Name_____

Reiki Master Manual
Including
Advanced Reiki Training

by
William Lee Rand

First Edition, October 2003, Revised Edition, June 2012

International Center For Reiki Training
21421 Hilltop St., #28, Southfield, MI 48033
Ph. (800) 332-8112, 248-948-8112, Fax 248-948-9534
email center@reiki.org, website www.reiki.org

Notice to Prospective Students

The ideas and techniques described in this manual are for Reiki students. They are not meant to be an independent guide for self-healing. If you have a health condition and intend to use Reiki, please do so under the supervision of an enlightened medical doctor or other health care professional.

Usage

Use this manual for teaching combined ART/Master classes. A separate ART manual is available for teaching ART by itself.

Published in the United States of America.

Vision Publications
21421 Hilltop St. #28, Southfield, MI 48033
Phone (800) 332-8112, (248) 948-8112 Fax (248) 948-9534
E-mail center@reiki.org   Web site www.reiki.org

Printed on recycled paper.
Contains fibers from trees
grown in well managed forests.

Table of Contents

Forms and Resources

Introduction

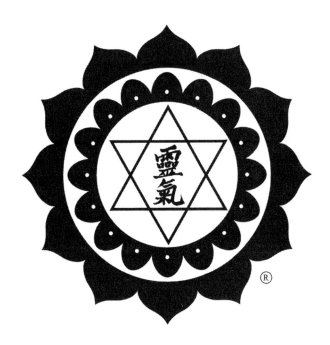

The Logo

The Japanese kanji in the center of the logo means Reiki, which is spiritually guided life energy. The upward pointing triangle represents humanity moving toward God. The downward pointing triangle represents God moving toward humanity. Because the two triangles are united, and balanced, they represent humanity and God working together in harmony. The inner sixteen petaled flower symbolizes the throat chakra or communication. The outer twelve petaled flower symbolizes the heart chakra or love. The complete logo represents Reiki uniting God and humanity in harmony through the communication of love.

The Logo is the Registered Service Mark of
The International Center for Reiki Training

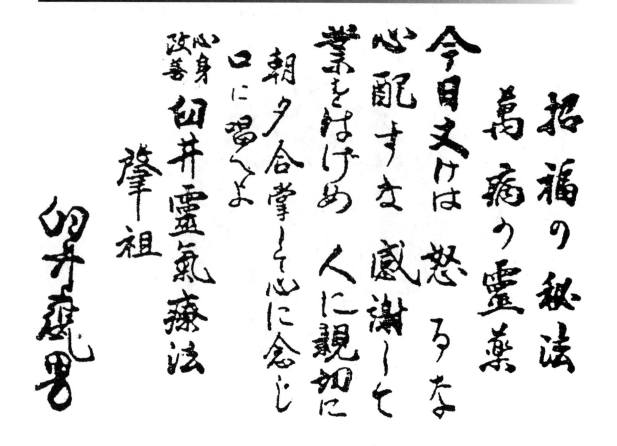

The Original Reiki Ideals

The secret art of inviting happiness
The miraculous medicine of all diseases
Just for today, do not be angry
Do not worry and be filled with gratitude
Devote yourself to your work and be kind to people
Every morning and evening join your hands in prayer,
pray these words to your heart,
and chant these words with your mouth
Usui Reiki Treatment for the improvement of body and mind

The founder. . . Usui Mikao

Introduction

It is always exciting when a Reiki student decides to become a Reiki Master. By deciding to take this step, you have started a process that will result in further enhancement of your skills as a healer. This will be a wonderful experience. There are many transformations that will take place within and around you. While some of these changes will be apparent to you, many will be beneath the surface of your everyday awareness yet will benefit your life and those around you just the same. If you have recieved this manual because you have signed up for the Master training, the positive changes associated with this process have most likely already begun. This is possible because your spiritual nature exists beyond time and space and began accepting special energies and preparing you for the class the moment you made the decision to attend.

The Japanese name for this class is *Shinpiden*, which means mystery teaching. The mystery is the mystery of our own existence—the mystery of life and consciousness. These qualities are boundless. No matter how much we experience them we will always find there is more, a next step, another doorway, a deeper level. And so the mystery is never completely solved but continues to become more fascinating and inviting as we heal more deeply and our awareness develops. Learning the Master symbols, experiencing the attunements and the class meditations and exercises along with the Reiki sessions we share with each other will further open you to this potential. The nature of this type of study—the

development of your connection to Reiki—evolves continually, healing you on deeper levels and developing your ability to channel ever more refined, effective and compassionate levels of Reiki healing energy. This is a joyous path that can continue on and on as long as you choose to remain a seeker.

Two Levels of Master Training
This class is an evolution of several traditions and forms of healing. The first segment of this class, Advanced Reiki Training (ART), developed out of changes that some teachers created after Takata Sensei passed on. She did not break the Master class into two levels, but taught only one level, which was the full Master training. After she passed, some of the Masters she trained began offering what they called 3A. This class was not the full Master training and was offered to those students who wanted the Usui Master symbol to use in their sessions but were not ready or not interested in being able to initiate and train others. This was a simple class that involved learning the Master symbol, receiving the attunement and taking time to practice giving sessions using the symbol. Those students who wanted to teach would later go on to take 3B, which included training on how to give the attunements. When I started teaching in 1989, I planned to teach a similar two-tiered format, but I added a number of additional techniques to both levels. These techniques give students additional healing skills. They were developed by following inner guidance and combining techniques and understanding from other healing methods with which I

was familiar. The Reiki grid is based on specific information about the energetic properties of crystals and how they interact with Reiki energy. It makes use of a crystal's ability to absorb the intention of the Reiki practitioner. One of the sitting meditations uses the Reiki symbols with Yantra meditation; another combines the Power symbol with the Microcosmic Orbit meditation practiced in Qi Gong and Taoism. The moving meditation is a synthesis of the principles of Qi Gong, Reiki symbols, Reiki energy, and affirmations. Aura Clearing (Psychic Surgery) draws its effectiveness from shamanism, Neuro-Linguistic Programming (NLP) and Reiki.

The Origin and Development of Usui Reiki

Usui Sensei received the gift of Reiki in March 1922 during a meditative experience on Kurama yama, a sacred mountain north of Kyoto.[1] At this time all he received was the healing energy of Reiki. Realizing its value, he was inspired to use it to help family members and others in need of healing. In April of the same year he opened a Reiki clinic in Harajuku, Aoyama, Tokyo and also started a healing society called the *Usui Reiki Ryoho Gakkai* (Usui Reiki Healing Art Society).[2] Through its use, he came to a deeper understanding of Reiki and over time developed many healing techniques to facilitate its use. These include: *Gassho* meditation, *Byosen scanning*, *Reiji ho, Gyoshi ho, Koki ho, Kenyoku*, and *Enkaku Chiryo*. He also developed a method of teaching Reiki and wrote a small manual for his students called the *Reiki Ryoho Hikkei* (Reiki Healing Art

Handbook).[3] Training sessions were held at the *Gakkai* several times a month and at each meeting *Reiju Kai* (attunement sessions) were given to each student. His training included: Shoden (first level) in which the student practiced *Gassho* meditation, gained the ability to give Reiki to oneself and to family members and perfected *Byosen* scanning, which he considered to be the basis of Reiki practice; *Okuden* (second level) in which the student became more competent with all methods of giving Reiki, learned the three Reiki symbols and began giving Reiki sessions to others; and *Shinpiden* (mystery level) in which one became a teacher.[4] (Neither Usui Sensei nor Hayashi Sensei made use of a fourth or Master symbol.)[5] Usui Sensei continued to teach and practice Reiki and trained twenty *Shihan* (teacher), each having the same ability to practice and teach as himself.[6] He passed through transition March 9, 1926.[7]

Chujiro Hayashi

Hayashi Sensei may have been one of the last Reiki students Usui Sensei trained as a *Shihan*. Hayashi Sensei was also a medical doctor and had been an officer in the Navy. Usui Sensei gave Hayashi Sensei the assignment of further developing the Usui system from the perspective of a medical doctor. Hayashi Sensei remained a member of the *Gakkai*

---

[1] Tadao Yamaguchi, *Light on the Origins of Reiki, A Handbook for Practicing the Original Reiki of Usui and Hayashi* (Wisconsin: Lotus Press, 2007), 62.

[2] Inscription on the Usui Memorial stone, Saihoji temple cemetery, Tokyo.

[3] Frank Arjava Petter, *The Original Reiki Handbook of Dr. Mikao Usui* (Wisconsin: Lotus Press, 1999).

[4] William Rand, "Interview with Hiroshi Doi, Pt. I," *Reiki News Magazine* (Summer 2003). Doi is a member of the Usui Reiki Ryoho Gakkai.

[5] This information is validated by the research of Hiroshi Doi, Tadao Yamaguchi, Hyakuten Inamoto, and Frank Arjava Petter.

[6] *Reiki News Magazine* (Spring 2011), 18. Photo of Usui Sensei and the twenty Shihan.

[7] Inscription on the Usui Memorial stone, Saihoji temple cemetery, Tokyo.

at this time, but opened a Reiki clinic and school called *Hayashi Reiki Kenkyu Kai* (Hayashi Training Institute), which was separate from the *Gakkai*. In his clinic he carried out the assignment given to him by Usui Sensei and this resulted in the development of a new style of Reiki *Ryoho*. The new style contained the same energy lineage going back to Usui Sensei and many of the same techniques, such as *Byosen* scanning, but also contained new methods developed by Hayashi Sensei. These included a new system of *Reiju kai*, a specific hand placement system for various illnesses and conditions (which were to be used only if the student couldn't find the areas needing Reiki using *Byosen* scanning) and developed a handbook called *Reiki Ryoho Shinshin* (Guidelines for Reiki Healing Method).[8] Also, in the original Usui method, the client would sit in a chair and receive a session from one practitioner, but Hayashi Sensei had several practitioners simultaneously give Reiki to one client with the client lying on a Reiki table. When he was traveling outside Tokyo, Hayashi Sensei developed the method of teaching *Shoden* and *Okuden* together in a five-day class with two to three hours of class time per day.[9] After Usui Sensei's transition, Dr. Hayashi left the *Gakkai* and became independent.[10]

Hawayo Takata

Takata Sensei enrolled in Hayashi Sensei's school in Tokyo in 1935. Her *Shoden* training took four days. After this she completed a yearlong internship at the clinic giving Reiki sessions to clients who came to the clinic and also making house calls. At the end of her internship, she was promoted to *Okuden*.[11] Based on entries in her diary it is likely she began *Shihan* training in Japan and according to her Reiki certificate it was completed in Hawaii in 1938.

Takata Sensei established a Reiki practice in Hilo the following year, just two years prior to the 1941 Japanese attack on Pearl Harbor and the U.S. entry into World War II. This event created a conflict for her, as she was trying to teach a Japanese technique at a time when most Americans viewed everything Japanese in a negative light. This may be the reason she changed the history of Reiki in an effort to make it appear more Western. However, in addition to changing the history, she also simplified the way she taught and practiced Reiki, omitting much of what she had learned from Hayashi Sensei. This included leaving out *Byosen* scanning and most of the other healing methods developed by Usui Sensei. She created a new method of giving Reiki sessions, based on what she called a foundation treatment. This involved a set of eight hand positions that covered the abdomen, neck and head.[12] The legs and feet were not treated. She also said that Reiki was an oral tradition and in most of her classes didn't allow students to take notes or tape record and did not provide a class workbook or handouts.[13] While this is generally true,

[8] For a translation of this handbook, please see William Lee Rand, *Reiki, The Healing Touch: First and Second Degree Manual* (Southfield, MI: Vision Publications, 2011).

[9] Tadao Yamaguchi, *Light on the Origins of Reiki, A Handbook for Practicing the Original Reiki of Usui and Hayashi.* (Wisconsin: Lotus Press, 2007), 28.

[10] William Rand, "Interview with Hiroshi Doi, Pt. II," *Reiki News Magazine* (Fall 2003).

[11] Fran Brown, *Living Reiki, Takata's Teachings* (California: LifeRhythm, 1992), 29–30.

[12] John Harvey Gray and Lourdes Gray with Steven McFadden and Elisabeth Clark, *Hand to Hand, The Longest-Practicing Reiki Master Tells His Story* (Gray, 2002), 93.

[13] "Mrs. Takata Speaks," audiotape. This was also explained to me by Bethal Phaigh in 1981 when I took Reiki I from her.

she didn't always teach the same way and in at least one class she allowed her students to take notes and provided handouts.[14]

While it is unfortunate that Takata Sensei left out so much of what Usui Sensei originally taught, it's important to note that the style of Reiki she developed is effective. Because of this it is appropriate that we honor her as an innovator. In addition, without Takata Sensei, Reiki would have been lost to the West, as after World War II, the *Gakkai* became a closed organization, making it difficult for even the Japanese to learn Reiki. Because of Takata Sensei, Reiki continued to be available and has spread all over the world.

This brief history of Reiki is based on the latest verifiable facts. It is considerably different than the history originally taught by Takata Sensei. Rather than the system Takata Sensei taught being the unaltered method taught by Usui Sensei as she had claimed, we find that it is actually a new system she developed. And in fact we can see that from the beginning, Reiki has been a system that had been frequently modified by Usui Sensei, Hayashi Sensei, and Takata Sensei as a means of improving it.

Usui/Tibetan Reiki

Takata Sensei required all the Masters she trained to charge a fee of $10,000 for the Master level. She taught that this was a required fee, and if you did not charge this fee, then you would not be teaching Usui Reiki. The fee wasn't based on the length or quality of training

she provided, as no apprenticeship was included. The actual length of her Master training has not been documented by any of her Masters, except for Bethel Phaigh, who reported receiving both Level II and Master within a few days.[15] However, my conversations with a few of her Masters indicate in at least some cases her Master training lasted only a few days. According to Phagh, the high fee was to instill respect for the Master level. However, the high fee, along with the tendency of Takata Sensei's Masters not to teach many other Masters, was causing Reiki to spread very slowly.

Iris Ishikuro was one of Takata Sensei's Master students and Iris also had other training as a healer. She was involved with the Johrei Fellowship, a religion that includes healing with energy projected from the hands. She had also learned another kind of healing from her sister, who worked in a Tibetan temple in Hawaii. After Takata Sensei passed in 1980, Iris decided that she would follow her own inner guidance and teach for a more reasonable fee. As far as I know, she was the only one of Takata Sensei's twenty-two Masters who did this. The others continued to charge the high fee for Mastership.

Iris trained only two Masters. One was Arthur Robertson and the other was her daughter, Ruby. She asked them to always charge a reasonable fee. Ruby decided not to teach Reiki. However, Arthur Robertson did begin teaching in the mid-1980s. The reasonable fee allowed many more students to become Reiki Masters. He began giving Master trainings with ten to thirty students in

---

[14] William Lee Rand, "Takata's Handouts," *Reiki News Magazine* (Summer 2009), 58. This article contains the handouts and notes taken during one of her classes.

[15] Marianne Streich, "How Hawayo Takata Practiced and Taught Reiki," *Reiki News Magazine* (Spring 2007), 17.

each class. Those that Robertson taught trained others and the number of teaching Reiki Masters quickly increased.

Because Iris Ishikuro ignored the price restriction that Takata Sensei had placed on Reiki, she became the pathway through which Reiki would spread more quickly and eventually be passed on to people all over the world. In light of this, it is likely that the majority of Reiki people in the world have their lineage going back through Iris Ishikuro.

Arthur Robertson had also been a teacher of Tibetan shamanism and had learned a healing method that made use of several symbols and an attunement-like technique called an empowerment. This method had similarities to Usui Reiki. After becoming a Reiki Master, he developed an alternative method of Reiki that was a combination of the Tibetan style of healing and Usui Reiki. The parts from Tibetan shamanism were the use of two Tibetan symbols—with one being used as a Master symbol—and the Violet Breath. It also incorporated the use of the three symbols from the *Okuden* level of Usui Reiki. He called this system Raku Kei.[16] Robertson taught both the Takata-style Usui system and *Raku Kei,* teaching them separately in different classes.

My first Reiki Master teacher, Diane McCumber, learned Reiki from Arthur Robertson and was taught both the Takata-style Usui system and the *Raku Kei* system. While I learned both from her in March 1989, she mainly taught the *Raku Kei* system. Later the same year,

I was also taught the Usui system by Marlene Schilke, who had also learned from Arthur Robertson.

As time went on, many of my students wanted to learn both systems but didn't want to take both classes and asked me if I could combine them. After meditating on this I realized that it could be done. I experimented and eventually developed the system I began calling the Usui/Tibetan system of Reiki. It simplified the process of attunements for Reiki I by using the one-attunement system from *Raku Kei.* When I combined the two attunement systems, I included all the steps and symbols used in the four-attunement system of Usui Reiki I. This made it a powerful, yet simple system that was easy to learn. However, the original Usui system of attunements as taught by Takata Sensei is also included in this manual, so anyone taking the Master training can choose to use either the Takata-style Usui system of attunements (that includes the four-attunement method for Reiki 1) or the Usui/Tibetan method of attunements that requires just one attunement. In addition, a four-attunement method is also included in this manual for the Usui/Tibetan system.

Teaching Reiki I and II Together
Some students are also curious as to why I teach Reiki I and II together when some teachers insist they must be taught separately with a certain period of time between them. There are many benefits in teaching them together, including the fact that the students leave class with greater healing skill and ability.

Actually, teaching Reiki I and II together is more traditional then what many have been told. I learned Reiki I in 1981 and since that time have spoken with many people

[16] Personal interview with Arthur Robertson at the Spiritual Frontiers Fellowship during the summer of 1989.

9

In who took classes from Takata Sensei and some who sponsored her classes. From this information it is clear that she sometimes taught Reiki I and II back to back or as part of the same class or taught them with just a few days in between.

In 2001, I attended a Reiki I and II class in Japan taught by Chiyoko Yamaguchi Sensei. She was in her eighties at the time. She had received her Reiki training from Hayashi Sensei. She came from a Reiki family, and Hayashi Sensei came to their home once a year to hold Reiki classes. At these classes, she was his assistant. She taught in the same style that she was taught by Hayashi Sensei—and she taught Reiki I and II together in one five-day class as this is how Hayashi Sensei taught when he was traveling. This information is further verified in a book written by her son, Tadao Yamaguchi.[17]

We can see from these examples that teaching Reiki I&II together is a traditional option. However, organizational skill and experience are required if one is to do a good job when teaching them together. Therefore, I recommend that for new teachers or for those who feel guided to do so, teaching them separately is also an option.

There are different ways one can approach the process of learning, practicing and teaching Reiki. The experience of the Japanese Samurai can shed light on this subject. In one Samurai tradition, the student was to study with just one teacher and to be loyal to that teacher and practice and teach exactly what had been taught. The purpose was to maintain the same style over many generations. Originally this method was taught in the oral tradition with no text to refer to.[18] The emphasis was so strong on teaching only the correct methods, teachers sometimes left out details they weren't sure were correct. Over time this tradition taught less and less and because of this, lost vitality and eventually died out.

However, there was another Samurai tradition in which the student studied with many teachers—first mastering what was taught by one teacher before going on to the next. This method placed an emphasis on understanding the essence of Samurai philosophy, which could more easily be perceived by comparing the various styles. Eventually the student developed his own style based on a synthesis of the many styles that had been learned. In addition, it was his responsibility to eventually add new methods based on experience. When it came time to teach, the Samurai would teach from a broad background of training and experience in which the essence was retained and passed on. This tradition had tremendous vitality and grew stronger over time.

This second Samurai tradition is the study and training method I had followed out of high school when I realized that metaphysics and healing were my passion and that I wanted to learn all I could about both. Over a period of 15 years or so I would join a particular school, or train with a teacher or take classes in a particular metaphysical subject until I became competent with what was taught. Then I'd go on to another school or teacher or class.

17 Yamaguchi, Light on the Origins of Reiki, 28.

18 Inazo Nitobe, Bushido, *The Soul of Japan* (Feather Trail Press, 1904), 11.

In this way I became proficient in many areas of metaphysical practice.

When I came across Reiki, I immediately became aware that it placed one directly in contact with the Source and that it was a healing method that embodies a higher level of consciousness than the previous healing methods I had studied. Eventually Reiki became my sole focus, and I studied and practiced it using the same intensity and methods as with my previous studies.

After taking Reiki I in 1981 and Reiki II in 1982, and becoming a Reiki Master in 1989, I decided to continue my training and take the Master class from a number of Reiki Masters. I learned the Usui/Takata style, the Raku Kei style, and several of the Japanese styles. I also sponsored Arjava Petter to teach his Japanese Reiki Technique classes in 1999 and 2000 in the U.S. and so had the great opportunity of thoroughly learning the Japanese Reiki healing methods that had been left out by Takata Sensei. In addition, I have studied the Japanese Reiki Techniques with Chiyoko Yamaguchi Sensei and her son, Tadao Yamaguchi Sensei, and also with Hiroshi Doi Sensei and Hyakuten Inamoto Sensei. This broadened my understanding of Reiki and helped me in many ways. (See my lineage chart on page 13.)

The Evolution of Reiki
One thing I came to realize from my training experience is that there is no limit to the possibilities offered by Reiki. As demonstrated by Usui Sensei and Hayashi Sensei, Reiki is something that can be developed. This is true for the techniques one uses to practice Reiki, but it is also true for the quality of the healing energy.

Reiki energy comes from an infinite source and because of this, regardless of how developed and evolved ones healing energy has become, one will always be channeling only a small portion of the potential healing energy that is available; it is always possible for the quality, effectiveness and benefit of one's healing energies to improve as well as what takes place in the attunements. Usui Sensei alluded to this when he said he wasn't at the top of the Reiki healing system, but one step below. It is also important to note that Jesus, who is by far one of the greatest healers we have information about, said that we could do everything he had done and even more.[19]

When a student first becomes a Reiki Master and begins teaching, he passes on the energies he has received from his teacher. However, if the new teacher continues to work on his or her own healing in a way that heals what can be called the "Reiki self" and in so doing creates greater alignment with the source of Reiki, the energetic frequencies channeled in healing sessions along with the energies passed on during the attunements will develop, taking on a higher, more refined and effective quality that is unique to that particular teacher.

As Reiki has continued to spread and develop, many different styles and qualities of Reiki have emerged. If a student is to cultivate an ever more refined and beneficial quality in his or her healing energy, it's important to carefully choose whom to study

---

[19] John 14:12 (NIV). "I tell you the truth, anyone who has faith in me will do what I have been doing. He will do even greater things than these, because I am going to the Father."

11

with. This process may be likened to properly furnishing a home. To do this well, one must choose furniture that is of the same or higher quality and similar style and that matches and complements the style one has. In this way a sense of balance and harmony is felt in the home. If our purpose is to develop the quality of our healing energy, it's important that we follow a similar process and carefully choose teachers who are teaching a style that is in harmony with our own and that will enhance what we already have.

It is fortunate that you are at this point in your Reiki training when you are receiving the ability to teach others. This is a glorious time when many new and exciting experiences are taking place. Therefore, it's important that you pay attention to what you are experiencing and be alert to the changes taking place within yourself so you can appreciate and savor this precious moment. May the love of Reiki heal and bless all you do.

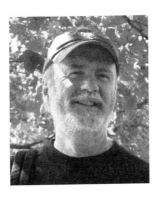

William Lee Rand
Usui Reiki Master Lineage

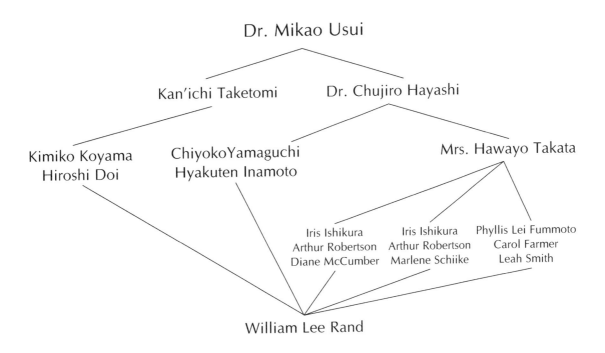

Dr. Mikao Usui

Kan'ichi Taketomi   Dr. Chujiro Hayashi

Kimiko Koyama   ChiyokoYamaguchi   Mrs. Hawayo Takata
Hiroshi Doi   Hyakuten Inamoto

                        Iris Ishikura   Iris Ishikura   Phyllis Lei Fummoto
                        Arthur Robertson   Arthur Robertson   Carol Farmer
                        Diane McCumber   Marlene Schiike   Leah Smith

William Lee Rand

William received Reiki I in 1981 and Reiki II in 1982 from Bethel Phaigh who received her master training from Mrs. Takata. In 1989 he received the master training from Diane McCumber and Marlene Schiike and in 1991 from Leah Smith. In 2002, he received the master training in Gendai Reiki from Hiroshi Doi and also in 2002 the Komyo Reiki training from Hyakuten Inamoto. In 2001 he took Reiki I&II from Mrs. Yamaguchi and her son Tadao in Kyoto, Japan. William has taught Reiki full time since 1989 in the U.S. and in countries all over the world. He is also author of *Reiki for a New Millennium* and also co-authored *The Spirit of Reiki* with Arjava Petter and Walter Lubeck. In 1994-95, he developed Karuna Reiki®. He is also founder and president of the **International Center for Reiki Training**, publisher of the *Reiki News Magazine* and the *Online Reiki Newsletter*. The Usui/ Tibetan style of Reiki which he teaches is a combination of Japanese and Western Reiki methods.

The Center Philosophy

- Honesty and clarity in one's thinking.
- Willingness to recognize prejudice in oneself and replace it with truth and love.
- Compassion for those who have decided not to do this.
- Speaking the truth without judgment or blame.
- Respecting others' right to form their own values and beliefs.
- Placing greater value on learning from experience and inner guidance than on the teachings of an outside authority.
- Basing the value of a theory or technique on the verifiable results it helps one achieve.
- Being open to results rather than attached to them.
- Taking personal responsibility for one's situation in life.
- Assuming that one has the resources to solve any problem encountered, or the ability to develop them.
- Using negative and positive experiences to heal and to grow.
- Trusting completely in the Higher Power regardless of the name one uses.
- Complete expression of Love as the highest goal.

The Center Purpose

- To establish and maintain standards for teaching Reiki.
- To train and license Reiki teachers.
- To create instructional manuals for use in Reiki classes.
- To encourage the establishment of Reiki support groups where people can give and receive Reiki treatments.
- To help people develop and use their Reiki skills.
- To encourage students to become successful Reiki teachers if they are guided to do so.
- To research new information about Reiki and to develop new techniques to improve its use.
- To openly acknowledge the value provided by all Reiki people regardless of their lineage or affiliation.
- To promote friendly cooperation among all Reiki practitioners and teachers toward the goal of healing ourselves and Planet Earth through the use of Reiki.

Tools & Techniques

Reiki Healing Process

After taking a Reiki class or even after a treatment, some people report experiencing physical symptoms such as runny nose, colds, diarrhea, stomach aches, aches and pains in the body including headache, fatigue, etc. These symptoms that sometimes (but not always) happen are caused by healing changes taking place in the body. If you have had traumatic experiences in the past, or been in a weakened or sick condition or have been operating at less than your highest level of health, toxins tend to accumulate in various tissues of the body. Even though the toxins are stored, they still create a burden on the healthy functioning of your system. When healing takes place, your system will begin operating on a higher level of efficiency and begin releasing these stored toxins. When this occurs, they enter the blood stream and then are eliminated by the lungs, liver, kidneys and bowel, through the skin and in other ways.

Another thing to consider is that if one or more organs have been operating at less than optimal health, the other organs in the body must compensate for them. When the weak or sick organs heal, not only do *they* change the way they have been operating, but so too must the ones that were compensating for the weakened ones. Because of this, many parts of the body go through a period of adjustment when healing takes place. And in the same way that a muscle that hasn't been exercised in a while will feel sore at first when it does begin to be used, many of your organs will also feel sore as they adjust to the new, healthier way of functioning.

The healing process can sometimes cause the uncomfortable symptoms mentioned above. These experiences are actually part of your recovery as you enter a more deeply healed state. This is sometimes called a "healing crisis" by some, but is actually a normal part of the healing process.

So when this happens, keep in mind that it is actually a good sign and indicates that deeper healing is taking place. Once the toxins have released and the body adjusts to its new level of health, you'll feel better than ever! Just continue to nurture yourself, release all negative feelings to the light, get lots of Reiki and allow your healing to complete. Drinking more water, taking cleansing herbs, and getting more rest can also be helpful.

Healing can also take place on higher levels, affecting the emotions, the mind and one's spiritual life. This higher level healing can manifest in various ways and can bring about changes in the way one's life is organized. When this first starts to happen, it can sometimes manifest as an increase in the pace of life. There may be many more things to do and it may also seem like there are many more loose ends that need to be taken care of. In addition, some report difficulties with others including negative feelings that they haven't had in a long time. These feelings are often connected to events that have happened in the past with family, friends or others. Sometimes one will have problems at work or with relationships or with one's marriage.

This kind of stress after a Reiki treatment or attunement is also an indication of deeper level healing. This sometimes takes place because of the fact that when people truly begin to heal, their lives are affected on levels deeper than the physical symptoms about which they were concerned. We are holistic beings and all the parts of ourselves are connected. If healing takes place in one area, it can affect all other areas to a greater or lesser extent; when the original problem starts to heal, other parts of the person's life may need to change also. When this happens, a major reorganization may be required.

As an example, if you have a money problem, often what needs to change goes beyond just getting a better job. There are usually deeper issues involved such as your attitude toward your parents, which in turn may be connected to issues of responsibility, discipline, learning, handling rejection, etc. When your money problem begins to heal, all these other areas may be affected also so that all the stored negative feelings you had toward them will be activated.

The healthy thing to do is to allow yourself to feel these feelings and then release them. All of your habits of thought, feeling and action connected to these things will most likely need to be reorganized. If you feel this happening, it is important to recognize the changes that are trying to happen and with wisdom and thoughtfulness, flow with the process and allow the needed changes to take place.

As was previously stated, a "healing crisis" does not always happen after a Reiki treatment or attunement, but when it does, it is important to understand what is happening so you can support its completion.

Whenever change takes place, even if it is good, a period of adjustment is necessary so that the various parts of your life that were connected to the problem area can get used to the healthy new conditions. During this period, events can be quite confusing, and it may seem as though things are getting worse. If this happens, it is a good idea to talk with your Reiki practitioner, teacher or counselor about what is happening to get feedback and gain a better perspective on your experience.

Sometimes a deeper level healing can be likened to getting new furniture for your home. During the process of removing the old furniture and bringing in the new, your home will look and feel disarrayed and uncomfortable. Cobwebs and dirt may appear that you weren't aware were there. If people came to visit not knowing you are getting new furniture, they might think you were a poor housekeeper, and they may not feel comfortable in your home and want to leave. However, after the dirt and cobwebs have been cleaned up and the new furniture is in place, your house will look and feel better than ever and everyone will notice and appreciate the improvements that you've made.

It is the same way with personal healing; things may become confusing and uncomfortable before your healing is complete. However, after things settle down, it will be clear that important improvements have been made. You will feel much better and your life will be healthier. So be aware; if you are experiencing any of these uncomfortable things, it is likely that major healing is taking place and that soon your life will be healthier and filled with greater clarity and joy.

Reiki Moving Meditation

Your state of mind has much to do with your ability to accomplish goals and deal with the challenges of life. Being in a resourceful state of mind is a necessity if you want to achieve the best results. However, there may be times when you have an important task to do and do not find yourself in a positive state of mind. At these times, it is important to have a technique to help you release any negative feelings and bring in strong, healthy energies to help you accomplish your tasks.

There are many ways to influence your state of mind and one of the most powerful is through the use of the body. There is a direct connection between the mind and the body. Your state of mind is directly affected by your posture and the subtle energies employed in the way you use your body. Therefore, you can change your state of mind by directing your body to move in a positive, resourceful way. This is why dance, exercise and posture can be deeply healing when used with this understanding. If you are not feeling resourceful, move like someone who is resourceful and soon your state of mind will shift.

This *Reiki Moving Meditation* integrates Reiki energy more directly into the physical body. It is similar to a Tai Chi or Qi gong exercise, and incorporates Reiki energy along with affirmations and physical movement. This exercise helps anchor Reiki into the aura and physical body, creates a strong connection with the earth, heals the lower chakras, helps you become more centered in your own power and brings mental clarity.

Our purpose in living on the earth is to bring our spiritual consciousness, which is our true nature, completely into the body. This exercise causes this to happen.

Follow These Steps

1. Start with your feet about shoulder width apart and your knees slightly flexed. Draw several Reiki symbols on your hands, such as the Usui Dai Ko Myo and the Choku Rei or any other Reiki symbols you feel guided to use.

2. Then bring your hands together about 6" in front of your heart and about 8" apart. Think of Reiki and meditate on the Reiki energy developing and flowing between your hands. You may feel vibrations in and around your hands or even see wavy lines of energy flowing between your hands as the energy builds. See drawing 1.

3. After meditating on Reiki for a few minutes and feeling its energy, move your hands straight up over your head. Then turn you palms outward. Move your arms around slowly in a circle, and bring them back to where you started in front of your heart. Note that moving slowly and placing your attention on how the space you are moving through feels increases the effectiveness of this exercise. See drawings 2–6.

4. As you bring your hands back up in front of your heart, take in a deep breath. Then while breathing out, motion your hands down toward your feet and the earth and imagine sending the energy down through your legs and feet and deep into the earth. Imagine you can actually feel and see it going down into the earth. See drawings 7–8.

5. Steps 3–4 above are just the physical movement. These steps are repeated so it

is important to practice this several times to get the feel of it. Remember to do this movement with a feeling of confidence and power.

6. Now repeat steps 3–4 and while moving your arms around in a circle, chant "Dai Ko Myo" one time out loud. (If others will hear you, then simply chant it silently.) Start the chant as you move your hands downward and around and end it as they come back in front of your heart. Then motion the energy downward as described in step 4.

7. Repeat this entire process three times.

8. Now repeat the process substituting a new chant. This time say, "I establish my divine presence on earth." Repeat this three times.

9. Repeat steps 6 and 7.

10. Then do the entire process again using this chant "I accomplish my divine purpose on Earth," repeating this three times.

11. Now do the entire process using "Dai Ko Myo" again, doing this three times just as you did the first time.

This is one set. Do as many sets as you want. This exercise is very grounding, and energizing. It will help you become more centered in the power of Reiki. Do it before giving a Reiki session or before teaching a class. Do it before any important event. Do it when you get up in the morning to start your day or at any time you feel the need for more confidence and personal power. With practice you will find this a powerful way to enter a resourceful state of mind whenever you want.

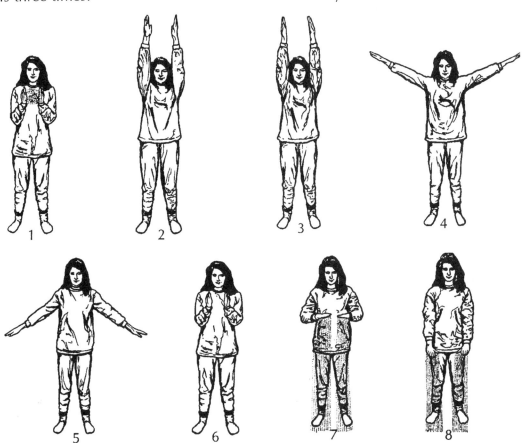

Reiki Meditation—Part One

Bringing In The Light

Reiki meditation works best if done every day and if done in the morning; however, you can also do it whenever you have the time. Twice a day is that much better. This is a very powerful meditation combining all the value of other types of meditation such as Transcendental Meditation plus the healing power of the Reiki energies. It can bring physical relaxation, mental clarity including improved ability to visualize, clairvoyance, enhanced healing skills, and the expansion of consciousness. It can also be used to solve problems and achieve goals, and it has the amazing tendency to surround all the areas of concern in your life with a soft white Reiki mist! Its value increases with regular use.

1. Sit quietly in a comfortable position with your hands on your legs or other part of your body, breathing slowly and deeply with your eyes closed as you think of Reiki.

2. Draw the Usui Dai Ko Myo in front of you using the whole hand with fingers together visualizing white or violet light coming from your fingers or the palm of your hand.

3. Hold the image of the symbol in your mind in front of you and repeat Dai Ko Myo three times. Say it out loud if no one will hear you or to yourself if others are around. Hold the visual image of the symbol steadily in your mind for several minutes and up to ten minutes. You may use a clock or watch and briefly open your eyes to check the time when you sense it is up. Do not worry if you find your mind has wandered away from the image or if you start thinking about other things. If you discover this has happened, do not berate yourself. Simply direct your mind back to the image. As you continue this practice each day, your ability to hold the image steadily will strengthen. If you have trouble visualizing, do the best you can. If you cannot visualize at all, and repeated attempts have not brought improvement, draw the symbol on a piece of paper or use the image in this manual; focus on it in the same way with your eyes open and relaxed. After a while, experiment with closing your eyes and retaining the image.

4. When you are finished meditating on the symbol, imagine it moving up into a field of light above you and bring your attention back in front of your eyes.

5. Repeat steps 2–4 with Choku Rei, Sei heki and the Hon Sha Ze Sho Nen.

6. Next imagine the symbols above you in a circle. Then imagine the circle of symbols descending down around you. Hold this image a few minutes and feel the energy of the symbols being absorbed into your energy field.

7. After meditating on the symbols, you will be centered and charged with creative healing energies. You can end the meditation now by going to steps 10 and 11 or you can continue with part two where you will be able to send Reiki to the projects and challenges of the day, actualize your goals and help or heal others at a distance.

Reiki Meditation—Part Two
Manifesting Goals

8. State your goal out loud or to yourself, create a picture of it in your mind to represent the goal accomplished and visualize the four Reiki symbols around it. Hold this image in your mind for several minutes or longer with the thought and feeling of accomplishment. Do this for each goal or project or to send help or healing to others. When you are finished with the image, state: "If this be possible within Divine love and wisdom, then let it be so." Then send the image up to the field of light overhead and place it within the other Reiki symbols with a feeling of fulfillment. Accept the idea that the process is complete and that your goal has been established. Believe this to be true, and then completely release it from your conscious attention.

If you are not a visualizer, simply write out the goal or healing on a piece of paper stating that it has been achieved along with the four Reiki symbols drawn in light and hold it between your hands accepting the idea that it is surrounded with light.

9. If you have a Reiki grid, use this time to charge your master crystal, which you would have been holding under your right hand during the Reiki meditation. Hold it between your hands and channel Reiki into it as well as projecting the four Reiki symbols into it. Then, after you are finished with the Reiki meditation, charge your Reiki grid. (See pp. 26-27)

10. To finish the Reiki meditation, place your tongue on the roof of your mouth and focus on the area just behind your navel. Then draw Choku Rei down the front of your body with the spiral around the area just below your navel. Pat your stomach three times and repeat Choku Rei three times. Then hold your attention on this spot steadily for several minutes and up to 10 minutes or longer. This will release any excess buildup of energy in your head and store it in the power center.

11. Then while breathing slowly and deeply, slowly open your eyes.

The Reiki Grid

The mass awakening toward higher consciousness and personal growth, which started in the 60s, has continually gained momentum. As each of us continues to work on personal healing, not only do we contribute to our own well-being, but the influence that we have on those around us helps them to grow as well. This synergistic effect allows the pace of our improvement to quicken even more. As healers work on each other and share their skills, a higher level of possibility for all of us is created. It must be remembered that the universe is a limitless reservoir of possibilities. To improve your healing skills, an open mind and a willingness to try new techniques is necessary. The Advanced Techniques taught in this class can add great value to your healing work. This technique uses crystals in a grid formation to assist in our distant healing work.

Crystals and Continuous Healing

One thing necessary for Reiki to work is your intention. You must intend for Reiki to flow in order to start it flowing. This can be a conscious or an unconscious intention and is often accompanied by placing your hands on someone. Quartz crystal has the unique property of being able to absorb and hold thoughts and intentions. Because of this, it is possible to place your intention as well as your ability to transmit Reiki into a crystal so that the crystal will continue to send Reiki while you are doing other things. This is valuable if you have someone you are working on who is really in need of healing.

Each crystal has its own vibration and there will be some crystals that are available to you that are better suited for use in sending distant Reiki than others. So the first step is to choose a crystal that is appropriate to use with Reiki. This can be done using your intuition, through the use of a pendulum, with muscle testing, with Byosen scanning, or some other method of accessing your inner knowing. After you have chosen a crystal, or in some cases after the crystal has chosen you, it is often necessary to cleanse the crystal of any inappropriate energy it may have. You can check if this is needed using any of the methods mentioned above. If it is indicated that the crystal needs cleansing, then simply place it in a bowl of rock or sea salt making sure it is covered with salt. Then do Reiki over the bowl of salt asking that the crystal be cleansed and blessed for your intended use with distant Reiki. Then leave it for 24 hours. All vibrations will be removed and you will then have a completely neutral crystal. There are many other ways to clean a crystal such as placing it under running water, placing it in the ground outside so the sun and moon will shine on it, placing it in saltwater, smudging it or doing Reiki on it with the intention of cleansing it. Use the method that feels right for you and the crystal.

After it is cleansed, it will be necessary to charge it with Reiki. Simply hold it between your hands and draw the Hon Sha Ze Sho Nen over it and do Reiki on it intending that the crystal will be charged with your ability to send distant Reiki. You can also visualize any other Reiki symbols you use entering the crystal. Steadily hold the image of each symbol in the crystal. Include a prayer asking that an Illumined Being bless your crystal and your intention to help and to heal others through its use.

After this initial process of cleansing and blessing, your crystal will be ready for use. There are several methods you can use to send distant Reiki continuously through your crystal, but they are all very similar. Simply take a picture of the person or if you don't have a picture, you can write the person's name on a piece of paper. Then place the paper in your hand and place the crystal over it. Draw Hon Sha Ze Sho Nen over the crystal and picture or name and say Hon Sha Ze Sho Nen three times intending that a Reiki connection be established. You can also add any other Reiki symbols you feel appropriate at this time. Then place both hands over the crystal and picture or name and begin doing Reiki intending that it be sent to the person. While you are doing Reiki, intend that the crystal will absorb your ability to send distant Reiki and that it will send it continuously. After sending Reiki in this way for 10 to 20 minutes or so, or longer if you have the time, set the picture or name down and place the crystal on top. Draw out the distant Reiki symbol again over the crystal and picture or name and then draw out Choku Rei. As you do this, intend that Reiki will continuously flow to the person for as long as it is needed or is valuable. If you have done this with a loving purpose, Reiki will continue to flow to the person for many hours or even days if it is needed. It can also be helpful to reaffirm your intention each day by following the above steps again. This process can also be used with a situation or with goals. Just write out a description of the situation or goal on a piece of paper and follow the same steps.

The blessings that will come to those you send distant Reiki to using this process will be truly wonderful. Also, any goals or situations you send Reiki to will also be blessed with love, new guidance and accomplishment.

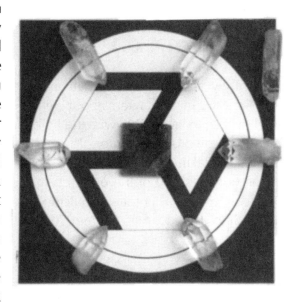

Creating a Crystal Grid for Continuous Reiki Healing

It is possible to create a grid or pattern using eight crystals and charge them with Reiki energy so they will continuously send Reiki to yourself or anyone whose picture or name you place in the grid. This advanced technique is more effective than the use of a single crystal and can be used to send Reiki to many people and situations at the same time. The beginning steps are similar to those necessary for using a single crystal. First, choose your eight crystals by asking for guidance in finding those that would work best in your Reiki grid. You will need six crystals for the outside part of the grid, one for the center and one to use as a master crystal. The center crystal can be a single or double terminated crystal, a crystal pyramid or a crystal ball or a crystal cluster. The master crystal needs to be a longer crystal like a laser or one with more of a yang or male type energy. It is also possible to use other kinds of crystals besides quartz. Always check with your pendulum or other method to be sure that any crystals or stones you choose will work and that they are willing to be used in the Reiki grid. Then cleanse them if they need it and charge them in the same manner as above.

Once they are charged, arrange the six outer crystals in a hexagram about eight to twelve or so inches across with the points, pointing toward the center. Place the central crystal in the middle with the point going between two of the outer crystals. The master crystal is placed outside the grid, off to the side. See diagram.

As you charge your Reiki grid with your master crystal, say a continuous series of affirmations or prayers such as: 'I charge this grid with light, with light, with light, to heal, to heal, to heal. I charge this grid with Reiki, with Reiki, with Reiki, to heal, to heal, to heal." You can also add: "I connect this Reiki grid to my highest spiritual guides to heal, to heal, to heal; I connect this grid to the power of God, to heal, to heal, to heal." Say this over and over also.

Then, once it is charged, anyone whose name or picture you place in the grid, will continuously receive distant Reiki. You can also place your goals or other situations on a piece of paper, and they will be blessed with Reiki also.

It will be necessary for you to charge your Reiki grid each day to keep it working. Doing this is like a meditation, as each time you charge it, you will feel like you are being charged with energy and becoming more focused as well. Because your picture is in the middle, you will also be receiving a continuous blessing of Reiki all day long.

If you go away and still want to keep your grid charged, take a photograph of your grid. Take the photo with you when you travel along with the master crystal. Then using Hon Sha Ze Sho Nen, connect with your grid through the picture and charge it using your master crystal. This will keep your grid charged and the picture itself will have energy around it and be very healing and protective for you to carry during your travels.

As we continue to receive additional training and to follow our inner guidance, not just for healing individual issues but also for the healing and guidance of our lives, we become more a part of the great transformation that is taking place on the planet. The upward flow of Reiki is growing continually stronger as more people on the planet are being attuned to this compassionate healing power. Do not hold back, but allow yourself to surrender completely to this upward flow of healing love. Then you will know what it means to truly be alive and to be free.

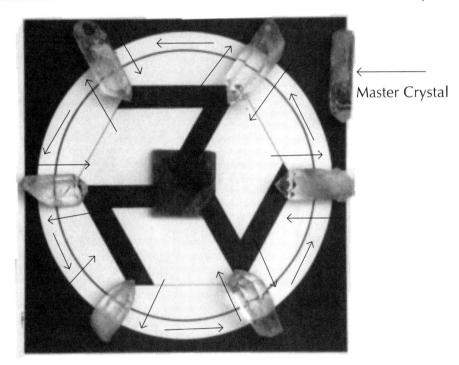

Master Crystal

The Reiki Grid

This is a Reiki Grid arranged on an Antahkarana symbol. Note that the six crystals are pointing toward the center. The master crystal is off to the side. An amethyst pyramid is at the center; however, you could use a single pointed crystal, a double terminated crystal, a cluster or a crystal ball. The arrows indicate the direction to point/move the master crystal when charging the grid. Move it from an outer crystal to the center, then back to the same outer crystal, then counterclockwise to the next crystal repeating the in and out motion and continuing around the circle. You may also be guided to move clockwise around the circle.

Quick Guide

1. Choose 8 crystals: 6 for the outer section, one central and one master. Use intuition, pendulum, muscle testing, scanning or simply choose those you like.

2. Cleanse them if needed. Then charge them with Reiki using all your symbols and especially Hon Sha Ze Sho Nen.

3. Place the 6 outer crystals in a hexagon pattern on a stiff piece of cardboard. Fix them in place using a small drop of rubber cement on the bottom of each crystal.

4. Place a picture of yourself in the middle with a positive affirmation on the back. Place the central crystal on top of the picture.

5. Charge your grid daily by first charging the master crystal with Reiki, then using it to charge the grid.

6. Place pictures or names of those needing healing or a written goal inside the grid, and they will receive continuous Reiki.

Aura Clearing

We all have dormant abilities inside ourselves waiting to be used. The ability to heal ourselves and each other is one of those abilities. It is simply a matter of claiming your power and developing the skill to use it. Aura Clearing (Psychic Surgery) is a tool that allows you to take charge of your inner power and use it to heal.

I developed this Aura Clearing technique based on training I received from a Kahuna while living in Hawaii. I took a technique I learned from him and after meditating on it and asking for help from my guides, combined it with a technique from Neuro-Linquistic Programming and Reiki energy. This technique is easily learned in class with the help of a Center Licensed Reiki Master or other experienced Reiki Master. By carefully following these instructions, you will be able to do Aura Clearing on yourself or your clients with powerful results.

The main reason people are not in optimum health is because they attract or create blocks to the flow of life energy within themselves. These blocks are usually made of ideas, beliefs and emotions that are opposed to the person's maximum well being. They are usually created because of misunderstandings about how to get one's needs met in a healthy way. Blocks to life energy are made of byoki or negative ki and usually take on a particular shape and lodge themselves in or around the organs of the body or in the chakras or aura. These negative energy blocks can cause health problems as well as other difficulties in life. Once they are removed, the life energy returns to its normal, healthy flow and the person's health is restored. Aura Clearing can be used to release these negative energy blocks. This process can assist in the healing of any problem or difficulty including emotional difficulties, relationship problems, addictions, spiritual problems as well as <u>physical health problems</u>. It must be kept in mind that if a person has a physical or psychological problem, it is important for you to advise them to see a licensed health care provider and to let them know that the purpose of your session is to work in conjunction with regular medical or psychological care.

Aura Clearing can be done by itself or in conjunction with a regular Reiki session, with Aura Clearing being done first or even during a regular session. You can also do this technique on yourself. (This type of Aura Clearing (Psychic Surgery) works with the energy field in and around a person. It does not actually cut open the body or remove physical tissue as is done with psychic surgery in the Philippines and other places.)

Steps

The first step is to give the cause of the problem an identity. This will allow the client and practitioner to focus directly on the cause and release it. Giving the problem an identity can be very healing in itself as it allows one to bring the cause into awareness where it can be dealt with. This involves finding the location of the block and deciding what it looks like.

1. Ask the client to think about the issue they would like to have healed. Note that it is not necessary for them to tell you what the issue is, just for them to think about it. This confidentiality can be very

28

helpful for many clients as some issues are so sensitive that the client may not want to let anyone know about the issue.

2. Ask the client to close her/his eyes and meditate on the issue. Ask this specific question: "If the cause of this problem were to exist in a part of your body, which part would it be in?" This is often easy, as the client will feel tension or pain in an area of the body whenever she/he thinks about the issue. Remind the client that if they are working on a physical issue, the cause may be located in area other than where the physical symptoms are located. If the client has any difficulty choosing an area, just ask the client to take a guess with the idea that there is no wrong answer.

3. Ask the client to imagine looking into the area they have chosen and ask this specific question: "If the cause of this problem had a shape, what shape would it have?" The shape is the shape of the negative energy that is causing or represents the problem. This could be any shape such as a cube, a sphere, a pyramid, a blob, broken pieces of glass, little spots or any other shape. Whatever shape chosen is will work; there is no wrong answer. If a physical organ needs healing, the cause will usually not look like the physical organ but will be a shape attached to the physical organ or close to it. It could also be somewhere else in the body or even in the aura. Sometimes there is more than one location. If that is the case, it is important to work with the most pronounced location first and then deal with the other(s) after that if they are still present.

4. Then ask this specific question; "If the shape had a color or colors, what would it be?" Then ask, "If you run your fingers over its surface, what texture would it have?" It could be smooth, slippery, rough or bumpy or some other texture. Then ask, "How heavy is it; how much does it weigh?" Then ask, "If what temperature is it." Then ask, "If it could make a sound, what sound would it make?" Remember that any answer is just fine and the client doesn't have to respond to all the questions.

After you get most or all of these answers, the cause will now have a nonverbal identity that the client will be consciously aware of. This process gives the client something to focus on. By having a location, shape, color, texture, weight, temperature and sound for the cause, the person will be more connected to the nonintellectual, energetic attributes of the cause and will be able to monitor its condition as you proceed with your healing work.

5. Ask the client if she/he is willing to completely let go of this cause and be healed now. Tell the client that you are going to send the problem up to God or the Higher Power. Ask her/him to focus on the shape and be willing to let it go. Also ask her/him to acknowledge and be willing to learn any lesson or receive any information necessary for the healing process to take place.

6. The client can be standing or sitting in a chair or lying on a Reiki table for the process.

7. Move behind the client or turn away from her/him so she/he can't see what you are drawing on your hands. Then draw the Usui Dai Ko Myo on both hands and clap them together three time repeating Dai Ko Myo to yourself three times. Do the same with Choku Rei. Draw Choku Rei down the front of your body for protection. Draw small Choku Rei's over each chakra to empower them. See drawing #1.

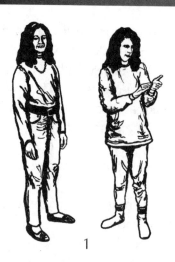

1

being, using your physical, emotional, mental and spiritual selves. It is done with complete confidence in your ability, knowing that Reiki is all powerful and that you will succeed. Note that it is your focused intention through which your guides will be able to work, so keep your intention clear and strong. This will be created in part by your posture, so when doing Aura Clearing, keep your posture confident, definite and clear so that there is no question about what you are doing.

8. Then extend your Reiki fingers. See drawing #2. This is done by grabbing hold of your fingers with one hand imagining they are made of taffy or some other malleable substance and imagine that you are stretching them out about 12" to 18" or so. As you do this, breathe in through pursed lips making an audible hissing sound. Do this several times. Then draw one Choku Rei on the ends of the extended fingers and tap them to affirm they are extended and have substance. Do this with both hands. Move your hands around imagining you can feel the extended fingers and the power they contain.

9. Aura Clearing is done with your full focus and intention. It is much like a martial art and done with your entire

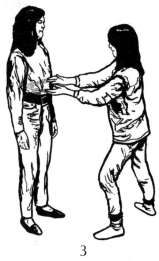

3

10. Say a prayer, either out loud or to yourself. Ask God, your fully Illumined Reiki guides, and the angels and archangels, to work with you to create the most powerful healing possible. Ask that the healing take place within Divine love and wisdom so that the highest good is created for all concerned.

11. Ask the client where the cause is located in the body and what its shape, color, texture, weight, sound etc. is. Ask her/him to focus on the area and be willing to let go of the shape and be healed. Draw Choku Rei over the area where the block is located.

12. Stand in a powerful position and using the full strength of your total

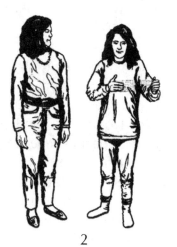

2

being, imagine you are reaching in and grabbing the negative energy with your

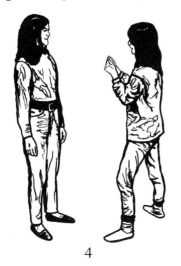

4

extended Reiki fingers, pulling it out and sending it up to God (or to the creative source of the Universe). Do this with physical, emotional, mental and spiritual intention—the full strength of your being. See drawings 3–5. You may actually be able to see the negative shape or you may be aware of it in some way, although it's not necessary to see or be aware of it for this technique to work. But if you are aware of it, use your perception to guide you in how you pull it out.

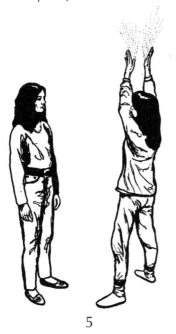

5

13. When you pull the negative energy out, breath in vigorously through partly closed lips, making an audible sound, and when you release the negative energy up to God, breath out vigorously making an audible sound. When using the breath in this way, imagine you are breathing the negative energy into your hands with it stopping at your wrists and not going any further. This will prevent you from pulling the negative energy into yourself.

14. Do this process over and over up to five to ten times or more—reaching in, pulling out the shape, and sending it up to the light.

15. After continuing for a minute or so, stop and ask the client how she or he feels and ask this specific question: "What does the shape look like now?" The shape may get smaller or change color or get lighter. These are all signs that the process is working.

16. If the shape doesn't seem to be getting smaller or isn't changing in some way or if it gets smaller for a time and then stays the same size, try pulling from different angles and sides of the area or try pulling from the other side of the body.

17. Continue with more sets of aura clearing stopping periodically to ask what the shape looks like now. Sooner or later he or she will say that the shape has completely gone. When this happens, ask him or her to look very carefully all around inside to be sure that it is completely gone and also to see if there is anything inside that doesn't belong there. If there is still some of the shape left or something that doesn't belong there continue doing Aura Clearing, periodically asking what the shape or energy looks like and continuing with this process until it is completely gone. When

the shape and any other negative energy is gone, you are done with this part.

The value of this technique is that as the practitioner, you do not have to be psychic or to have any awareness of the shape at all as the client will let you know what the shape looks like and about the progress you are making.

18. After the shape is gone, draw a Choku Rei over the area and give it Reiki to fill the area with light and complete the healing—see drawing #6. Then step back, make a karate chop in the air between the two of you to break any psychic cord(s) that may have formed. Also, retract your Reiki fingers by pushing them back into your physical fingers with your hand while making a blowing sound. You can follow this with a complete, hands on Reiki treatment if you have time.

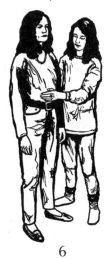

6

A Lesson May Need To Be Learned
Most psychic blocks can be easily removed using this process. However, if after doing several sets of Aura Clearing, you find that the shape has not changed or has changed very little, then it is likely that the cause of the problem has something to communicate to the client before it will be willing to leave. There may be a lesson the client needs to learn, and it may be necessary for the client to interact consciously with the cause in order for it to heal.

Follow These Steps
1. If you feel this is the case, draw Sei heki over the area and do Reiki there. As you do Reiki, talk directly to the cause and let it know that you respect the information it has to offer and that you are ready to hear what it has to say now. Ask it to tell you what it needs to do in order to heal. Then ask the client to focus on the shape and tell you whatever comes into his or her mind—even if it seems like nonsense. You can also start verbalizing whatever comes into your mind. At first it may not make sense, but ask the client to tell you if anything you say has any meaning or connection to the problem and if it causes any feelings or emotions to come up. Ask her/him to tell you if she/he gets any meaningful ideas about it too. You could get ideas like: "I need to let go of anger toward my mother." Or, "I feel guilty about the way I treated my younger brother when I was growing up. I need to forgive myself for what I did." Or, "I feel jealous about a friend who is successful, and I need to let go of this." You could get ideas like this, or something completely different or unique. However, let the client decide what feels right and what makes sense concerning what feelings come up and what needs to be done to complete the healing.

2. After you get an idea of what the client needs to do, ask if she/he would be willing to do it right now. If the answer is yes, then continue to do Reiki on the area and ask the client to take some time to focus on the shape and the issue and to process it—letting go of the anger, or forgiving him or herself or releasing the negative issues, etc. Ask the client to let you know when she/he feels complete with it.

3. After the client has done this and feels complete, ask her/him to look into the area and see if the shape is still there. It may be completely gone now, but if it is still there, proceed with more Aura Clearing. This time, the shape should release completely. Then draw a Choku Rei over the area and give it Reiki to fill it with light.

4. Step back, do the karate chop, and retract your Reiki fingers as described in step 18. You may want to follow Aura Clearing with a complete, hands on Reiki treatment.

One session is often all that is needed to completely heal an issue. However, some issues have more than one level, so the person may get some relief, but then experience more symptoms later as a deeper level of the issue comes up to be healed. If this is the case, simply do more Aura Clearing to heal the next level.

It is also important to know that as healing takes place, the person could feel other symptoms such as weakness, headaches, sadness or other feelings or symptoms as the body adjusts to the healing process and begins cleansing. This is sometimes called a healing crisis or recovery process (see page 17) and is part of the healing. To minimize this, it is important that the client drink more water, eats lightly and eats more cleansing foods, gets more rest and possibly uses cleansing herbs, as well as doing other things that facilitate inner cleansing.

This technique works. It is powerful and is easily learned by anyone willing to take the time to try it. All of our problems are within our ability to solve, and it is important to realize that there is always a higher purpose for everything in our lives. What we consider to be a problem may actually be an opportunity to learn and grow. Using inner guidance and developing new techniques that allow us to tap more deeply into our innate healing abilities are important parts of our growth process as spiritual healers. As we continue on further into the twenty-first century, there will be many opportunities to heal deeply and strengthen our connection to our true nature. Let us rejoice in the love and wisdom of life.

Quick Guide

1. Work with client to identify the location, shape, color, etc. of issue.

2. Prepare with symbols on hands, down front of body and each chakra, extend fingers.

3. Prayer.

4. Choku Rei over area on client you'll be working on.

5. Using hand motion, pull negative energy out as you breath in, and send it up to the light as you breath out. Do repeatedly.

6. Check with client periodically on what the shape looks like. Continue until shape is gone or has become positive.

7. If shape doesn't respond, a lesson or message needs to be communicated by the shape. Use Sei heki and ask for message. Use info for healing. Proceed with more Aura Clearing if needed.

8. Give Reiki to the area.

9. Break cord and retract fingers.

Reiki Master Meditation

This is a modified form of the Taoist Microcosmic Orbit meditation and is also a meditation used in Qi Gong. It works with the seven basic chakras including their back sides along with energy channels on the front and back of the body. The purpose of this meditation is to open and clear the chakras and create a clear pathway for energy to flow throughout your system. Usually it takes a student 4–6 months to open the energy pathways, but because Reiki has been added, namely the use of Choku Rei, the process is greatly accelerated and most find the energy pathways opening in the first or second session. This has been validated by one of my students who is a Qi Gong instructor and clairvoyant.

The master attunement brings in higher frequency energies that flow when you give sessions and when you give attunements. Higher frequency energies also enter your system during various kinds of meditation or other exercises for spiritual development. Clearing the chakras and the front and back channels will allow these energies to flow more easily and strongly. Doing this will also allow these higher energies to be fully assimilated and prevent problems caused by too much energy in the head or other parts of the body. It will also purify and/or release any negative energy from within yourself that you may have created or attracted. By circulating your energy, the negative energy is transmuted in the chakras as it passes through them and may also be released from the chakras. This happens automatically as you circulate it. This is a very worthwhile meditation that will create harmony and balance at the same time it brings

in greater levels of clarity and vitality. The channel on the front of the body is called the Functional channel and starts at the tongue and flows down the front side of the chakras to the root chakra at the Hui Yin point. The back channel is called the Governor channel and starts at the Hui Yin point and flows up the spine through the back sides of the chakras to the top of the head and ends at the top of the mouth. These channels are normally unconnected, but by placing the tongue on the roof of the mouth and lightly contracting the Hui Yin, the channels connect and form a circuit or what is called the microcosmic orbit, (note: this is not done until Part Two.)

Part One

1. To begin, sit with your feet flat on the floor. To enhance this meditation, you can also place one of the Antahkarana symbols under your feet. (see pg. 60-63) Choose the one you feel guided to use.

2. Draw the UDKM or the TDKM or both on your hands and place them on your legs intending that these energies will continue to flow throughout the meditation.

3. Say a prayer to God or to an enlightened being giving thanks for the healing and higher consciousness you are being sent.

4. Steadily hold an image of the Choku Rei on your solar plexus chakra. If thoughts arise, gently brush them aside and return to the image of the Choku Rei. Do not be disturbed if thoughts arise, as this is natural, but as soon as you realize thoughts are present, let them go and return your attention to the image of the

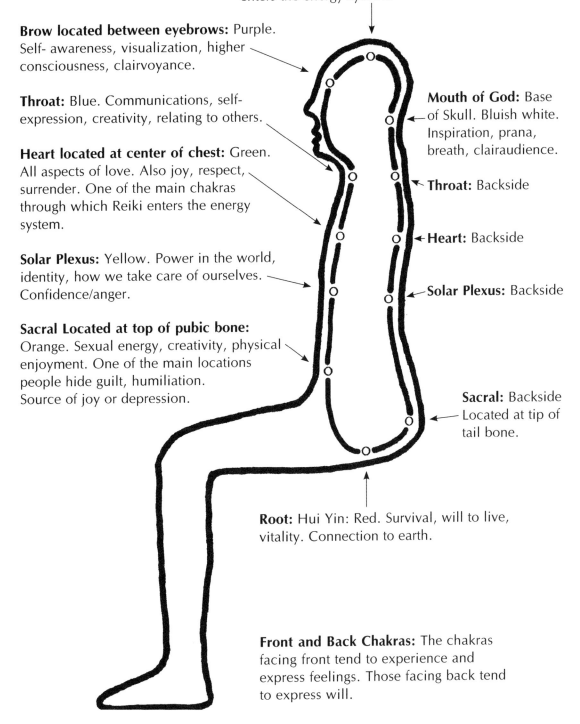

Crown: White. Spiritual Consciousness, connection to oneness and divinity. One of the main chakras through which Reiki enters the energy system.

Brow located between eyebrows: Purple. Self- awareness, visualization, higher consciousness, clairvoyance.

Throat: Blue. Communications, self-expression, creativity, relating to others.

Heart located at center of chest: Green. All aspects of love. Also joy, respect, surrender. One of the main chakras through which Reiki enters the energy system.

Solar Plexus: Yellow. Power in the world, identity, how we take care of ourselves. Confidence/anger.

Sacral Located at top of pubic bone: Orange. Sexual energy, creativity, physical enjoyment. One of the main locations people hide guilt, humiliation. Source of joy or depression.

Mouth of God: Base of Skull. Bluish white. Inspiration, prana, breath, clairaudience.

Throat: Backside

Heart: Backside

Solar Plexus: Backside

Sacral: Backside Located at tip of tail bone.

Root: Hui Yin: Red. Survival, will to live, vitality. Connection to earth.

Front and Back Chakras: The chakras facing front tend to experience and express feelings. Those facing back tend to express will.

Choku Rei on your solar plexus chakra. As you continue to practice this meditation, your ability to hold the image for longer periods of time without thoughts present will improve. By steadily holding this image in your mind, your mind will become calm, steady and powerful. The chakra will also open, clear and heal. Hold this image for approximately 2 minutes and up to 5 minutes.

5. Then move your attention down to the sacral chakra and repeat step 4. Continue this process with each chakra moving down to the root and then up the spine all the way around to the heart chakra.

6. As you proceed with this process, you may notice different sensations at each chakra point. You may feel heat, or coolness, see colors or images, etc. These are indications that healing or releasing is taking place. The important thing is to not be distracted, but continue to steadily hold the image. If you have any trouble visualizing, just do the best you can. As you continue, your ability to visualize will improve.

Part Two

1. After completing part one, place your tongue on the roof of your mouth and lightly contract the Hui Yin point, (see pp. 71).

2. Visualize a beautiful ball of white light in your solar plexus.

3. Then imagine the ball of white light moving down to the sacral chakra, then to the root chakra, then up the spine through the back sides of each chakra to the crown and down through the tongue and down the front. See this ball of light traveling around and around the energy pathway. The flow is always down the front and up the back.

4. Continue visualizing the ball of light traveling around the energy pathway for 10 minutes or more.

5. When you are ready to end the meditation, intend that the energy will continue to flow in this pathway. Then release the tongue and the Hui Yin point. Take a deep breath and open your eyes.

The value of this meditation increases with regular use. Over time you will find an increase in your ability to concentrate, increases in vitality, better sleep, improved health and ability to deal with stress, and most of all, it will increase the strength of your Reiki energy! I suggest you use it every day for at least two weeks to experience its value. Then decide if it is something you would like to include as a regular part of your development program. This meditation is available on the CD "Reiki Meditation."

Notes

Notes

Notes

40

Symbols

The Usui Reiki Symbols
by William Lee Rand

It is always important to know what a teacher's information is based on—that is, where it comes from. There has been a certain amount of information in the Reiki community that is based more on rumor than on verifiable facts. Because of this it is apparent that in some cases the information being passed on has become confused to the extent that non-Usui symbols are being called Usui symbols. The information for this article comes from the training I received starting in 1981 including training from three Reiki Masters who received their Masterships directly from Mrs. Takata, plus my continuing study and research into Reiki, which includes the exchange of symbols, attunements and important Reiki information with Reiki Masters from Japan and the West.

Usui Reiki symbols are sacred and are to be kept confidential. They are only revealed to those who are about to be initiated into the Second or Master Level of Reiki. The reason for this is explained later in this article.

Reiki symbols are an important and very interesting part of Reiki practice. They allow one to focus the energy of Reiki for specific purposes. (For a detailed explanation of what the symbols can be used for, see the book, Reiki, The Healing Touch.) There are a total of four symbols in the Usui System of Reiki as practiced in the West. Three are given in Reiki II and one in Reiki Master. There are other symbols that people are using, such as Raku, Johre, Lon Say etc., but they are not part of the Usui System.

Usui Reiki symbols are not as mysterious as they might seem. They are actually Japanese kanji, which means they are simply words from the Japanese language. Their names can be found in a Japanese/English dictionary. The first two symbols vary from this somewhat. While the words Choku Rei and Sei heki are Japanese, the Choku Rei symbol comes from Shintoism and is not kanji. Choku Rei means "By Divine decree." The symbol for Sei heki comes from the Sanskrit seed syllable hrih and also is not kanji. Hrih means love, but together, the words Sei heki mean "bad habit." Hon Sha Ze Sho Nen and Dai Ko Myo are Japanese kanji, both in their names and in the way they are drawn. Hon Sha Ze Sho Nen means "the origin of all is pure consciousness."

It is interesting to note that Dai Ko Myo can be found in The Encyclopedia of Eastern Philosophy and Religion and is translated to mean "treasure house of the great beaming light." It is said to be, "a Zen expression for one's own true nature or Buddha-nature of which one becomes cognizant in the experience of Enlightenment or Satori." This is quite a profound definition. Perhaps it is called the Master Symbol because it gives us direct connection to the Master Within, which is the real source of Reiki.

Recent information coming from Japan indicates that Usui Sensei and Hayashi Sensei used only three symbols, the three that are part of Okuden or Reiki II. The master symbol, Dai Ko Myo, was added to the system of Western Reiki sometime after Usui Sensei passed. We do not know for sure how it became part of Western Reiki. It may have been added by Takata Sensei, possibly with the help of Hayashi Sensei. The fact that Usui Sensei did not use a Master symbol has been verified by Hiroshi Doi Sensei, who is a member of the Usui Reiki Ryoho Gakkai, Tadao Yamaguchi Sensei, whose mother studied directly with Hayashi Sensei and Arjava Petter, who has done extensive research in Japan.

The above information indicates that the Usui Reiki symbols are not exclusive to Usui Reiki. They existed prior to their use in Reiki and were borrowed from other systems. It is likely that the three added by Usui Sensei came from his previous studies in religion and metaphysics.

The Reiki symbols are transcendental in their functioning. Whereas most symbols have an effect on the subconscious mind of the user, causing a change in one's internal state, the Reiki symbols access the source of Reiki directly and signal a change in how the Reiki energy functions, independent of one's internal state.

There are many ways to activate the Reiki symbols. They can be activated by drawing them with the hand, by visualizing them, or by saying the name, either out loud or to oneself. Intention is the main ingredient in activation, and it is possible with awareness to activate them by intention alone.

The power and effectiveness of the symbols come from the Reiki attunement that is given during a Reiki class. Before the attunement, the student is shown the symbols and given time to memorize them. During the attunement, the energies of each symbol come down and enter the student's mind/body, linking themselves to the appropriate symbol in the student's mind. Afterward, whenever the student uses the symbol, the same energies that they were linked to during the attunement are activated and begin flowing.

This process makes use of the stimulus/response mechanism, which is a dynamic part of the human mind. The Reiki symbol becomes the stimulus and the particular energy the symbol represents is the response. However, because the attunement is guided by the Higher Power, and functions at a higher level of awareness, the stimulus/response mechanism doesn't require the repetition normally necessary to establish a relationship between stimulus and response. It happens immediately.

The Reiki symbols have traditionally been kept secret. While secrecy is a way of honoring their sacredness, there are also metaphysical reasons for this. One of the benefits of keeping the symbols secret until just before the Reiki class and the attunement is to prevent them from becoming linked to non-Reiki energies. If a person is shown a Reiki symbol without the benefit of the attunement that empowers it, they may incorrectly believe they have Reiki and not bother to take a class, thus missing the real experience of Reiki and losing the benefit of its healing power. Furthermore, they may go on to practice Reiki sessions without having the real strength and effectiveness of the healing energy they would have had if they had taken a Reiki class, thus providing less benefit to those who come for healing. And if they teach what they call Reiki classes even though they don't have the authentic Reiki energy and the attunement to teach, they would be passing on something that really isn't Reiki, thus degrading the system of Reiki healing.

And even though Reiki symbols can easily be seen on the Internet by doing a search for "Reiki symbols," it's still important that students who have Reiki training and have been given the attunement for the symbols keep them private. This is because the spiritual beings who watch over Reiki and facilitate its flow do not want the practice of Reiki to be diluted by having people use the symbols who have not had the attunement for them. When they see someone sharing the symbols indiscriminately with those who are not about to take a class, they lose interest in supporting that person's Reiki. Because of this, his or her connection to the source of Reiki is weakened and their Reiki energy will not be as strong or effective as it would have been if they had continued to honor the secrecy of the symbols. However, there is no problem sharing the Reiki symbols with those who have already had that level of Reiki training.

Many have noticed differences in the way the symbols are drawn when compared to the symbols from other Reiki Masters. These differences are there for a number of reasons. First, it is known that Takata Sensei did not always draw the symbols exactly the same for every student she taught. After her transition, there was a meeting of the Reiki Masters she initiated. At the meeting they compared how their symbols were drawn. The Choku Reis of all the Masters present were basically the same. Sei hekis of the Masters had some

slight differences. However, Hon Sha Ze Sho Nens were quite different—especially with the strokes at the bottom. They did not compare their Dai Ko Myos. So, even at this early date, there were differences that apparently came from Takata Sensei herself. Perhaps she deliberately drew them differently to give a little distinction for each student or perhaps at other times, because of age or from having taught for over 30 years, she accidently drew them with some differences. Also, there are different ways to draw the Japanese kanji figures, and in fact, Takata Sensei did have two ways of drawing the Dai Ko Myo: One way was more of a flowing style, called "running hand," with the main difference found at the bottom part of the symbol, with two boxes containing an arrow and a Z. The other way she drew the Dai Ko Myo was in a printed or block style called "normal." However, both ways of drawing the Dai Ko Myo have exactly the same meaning.

So starting out there were already changes in the symbols from one student to another. Add to this the fact that in the early days of Reiki in the West, students were not allowed to make written copies of the symbols; they were required to keep them only in the mind. When it came time to pass them on, the teachers had to draw them from memory. Since few people have perfect memories, some changes were bound to occur. This process has continued over and over, thus allowing more changes to take place. What is surprising is that for most students, the symbols still look fairly close to the original. Additional note: The symbols used by Chiyoko Yamaguchi Sensei in Japan, who learned from Hayashi Sensei, are somewhat different than those taught by Takata Sensei.

Therefore, the question arises about whether there is a perfect or correct way to draw and visualize the symbols. From the above example, it can be seen that even those who learned directly from Takata Sensei did not draw the symbols in exactly the same way—leading one to believe that there must not be one perfect way to draw them. It has also been found that everyone who has received the appropriate attunement for the symbols has symbols that work. So the power of the symbols does not come from drawing them or visualizing them in one perfect way. It comes from the link that is made between the symbol the student receives in class and the attunement energies entering the student during the Reiki initiation. The correct way to draw the symbols is the way your Reiki Master drew them for you before you received the attunement, as it is the link between the symbol and the Reiki energy that takes place during the attunement that empowers the symbols. However, if you are teaching Usui Reiki, then it is your responsibility to make sure the symbols you are using are the same or at least similar to those used by Takata Sensei or Usui Sensei.

The Reiki symbols are a wonderful, simple way to connect to the Higher Power. Their use does not require that we be able to meditate or have years of spiritual practice. Their effectiveness comes to us by grace, which allows us to humbly accept the value we receive as a gift from the Creator. We are grateful for the efforts of Usui Sensei and all the others who have lovingly worked to make this system of healing available to us.

Kanji Symbols

The Reiki Distant and Master symbols come from Japanese kanji, which are actually characters from the Japanese language. The word kanji means Chinese characters and this is because China is where Japanese kanji originated. In fact the meaning of both Japanese and Chinese characters is very similar to the extent that Japanese and Chinese people can read and understand each other's written language. Each character can have different meanings depending on the context it is used in and how it is used in combination with other characters. Their use as Reiki symbols is in a very specific context and because of this, the meaning varies from the standard meaning listed in a dictionary. See the previous article for their meaning as Reiki symbols. Below are sections from the Japanese/English dictionary, *Essential Kanji*, by PG O'Neill.

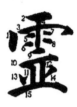

1299; 173/7. REI, RYŌ, *tama* spirit, ghost, soul
[LING² • I: in the heavens 1-8, lines 9-15 (cf. 998) of spirits]
亡霊 — *bōrei* — dead spirit, ghost
慰霊祭 — *ireisai* — memorial service

144; 84/2. KI, KE spirit ⌜rice 5-6; P*⌝
[CH'I⁴ • I: the vapour 1-4 rising from cooking
気持ち — *kimochi* — feeling, mood
天気 — *tenki* — weather

32; 37/0. DAI, TAI, *ō(kii)*, *ō(ki na)* big; *ō(i ni)* greatly ⌜P*⌝
[TA⁴ • D: a man with arms & legs spread wide;
大目に見る — *ōme ni miru* — overlook, let pass
大水 — *ōmizu* — flood

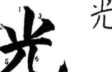

217; 42/3. KŌ, *hika(ru)* shine; *hikari* light, ray
[KUANG¹ • I: a torch 1-3 (= 15) carried by a man 4-6; P*]
日光 — *nikkō* — sunshine, sunlight; pn.
発光する — *hakkō suru* — radiate, emit light

58; 72/4. MEI, MYŌ, *aka(rui)*, *aki(raka na)* bright; *a(keru)* to dawn; *a(kasu)* pass the night, divulge
[MING² • I: sun & moon together; P*]
明日 — *myōnichi/asu, ashita* — tomorrow
明け方 — *akegata* — (early) dawn

本

本 20; 2/4. HON* book; unit for counting cylindrical
objects; *moto* source, origin
    [PEN³ • D & S: line at base of tree trunk; P*]
日本 — *Nihon* / *Nippon* (ir.) — Japan
六本木 — *Roppongi (← roku + hon + ki)* — pn.

者 56; 125/4. SHA, *mono* (dep.) person
    [CHE³ • I→B; P*]
目下の者 — *meshita no mono* — an inferior/junior
読者 — *dokusha* — reader

是 786; 72/5. ZE right, just
    [SHIH⁴ • R sun & P*]
是非 — *zehi* — right or wrong, without fail
是認 — *zenin* — approval

正 123; 1/4. SEI, SHŌ, *tada(shii)* correct; *masa (ni)*
exactly, certainly   ⌈right; P*]
    [CHENG⁴ • I: a foot 2–5 toeing the line 1, exactly
正月 — *shōgatsu* — the New Year, January   ⌈ior
正しい行ない — *tadashii okonai* — correct behav-

念 316; 9/6. NEN* thought, idea, wish
    [NIEN⁴ • R heart & P*]
残念 — *zannen* — regret   ⌈issue
記念号 — *kinen-gō* — commemorative number/

49

Notes

Hon Sha Ze Sho Nen

Sei heki

Choku Rei

Second Degree Usui Reiki Symbols
as drawn by Takata Sensei

51

The Usui Master Symbol

There are several ways to translate the meaning for the kanji of the Usui Master symbol. One translation is: "Great being of the Universe, shine on me, be my friend." *The Encyclopedia of Eastern Philosophy and Religion* lists a definition for this symbol as "Treasure house of the great beaming light," and states that it is "a Zen expression for one's own true nature or Buddha-nature, of which one becomes cognizant in the experience of Enlightenment or Satori."

Use of the Usui Dai Ko Myo in conjunction with Reiki creates a noticeably stronger channel between the Physical Self and the Higher Self. This allows more of the unlimited wisdom and power of God to manifest directly on the physical plane. It intensifies and focuses the Reiki energy, causing it to more firmly establish positive results in a definite, grounded and permanent way. And it protects the healing work that it does by preserving its value so that the healing effect takes place for a much longer time after it is used in a Reiki session.

All the qualities of Reiki, including the actions of the other symbols, are enhanced by the use of the Usui Dai Ko Myo. It seems to bring with it a greater feeling of wholeness, fulfillment and completion. It is very satisfying to feel its power flow through and around you whenever you use it in conjunction with Reiki. It is similar to Choku Rei in many ways except that it operates on a much higher frequency and brings into use a higher level of divine power. Once you have been attuned to use this symbol, it is valuable to use it first, before using the other symbols, as it will empower them. The Usui Dai Ko Myo can be used when giving Reiki sessions, and it can also be used to empower any other kind of healing, manifesting or personal transformation work. It can be used as part of a ritual and also in conjunction with physical movement. It can be used to bless and empower all activities! Let your imagination help you create new uses for it.

Try this any time after you have received the attunement for the Usui Dai Ko Myo. You can do this anywhere, even while driving. First think of Reiki. You do not have to have your hands on yourself, as Reiki will simply begin flowing out your hands regardless of what you are doing with them. Once you feel Reiki flowing, begin chanting Dai Ko Myo three times either out loud or to yourself, followed by: "I establish my divine presence on earth," three times. Do this over and over allowing yourself to feel the power you are creating.

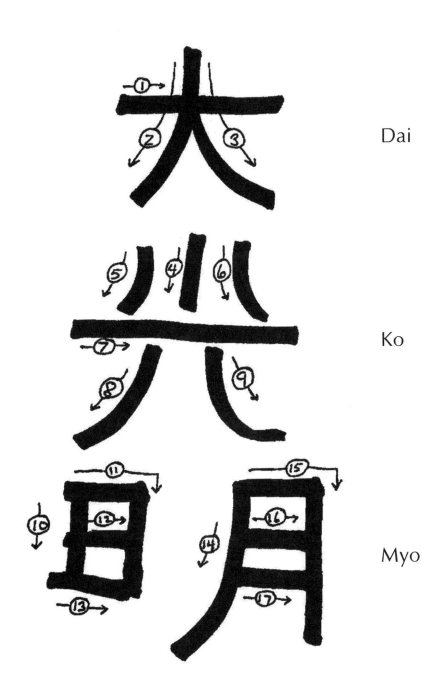

Dai

Ko

Myo

Usui Dai Ko Myo
Reisho Style

Tibetan Dai Ko Mio

The energy of this symbol is very similar in nature to the Usui Dai Ko Myo explained on pages 52. However, many feel it has a gentler way of healing and yet is more powerful. It is used in the attunement process as part of the Violet Breath explained on pages 72. It can also be used as a treatment symbol. It creates a very holistic healing energy that has a higher vibration than the Reiki II symbols. It assists in healing a wider range of conditions more quickly and at greater depth. It has also been found to be useful in pulling out negative energy and because of this, it can be added to the symbols used in Aura Clearing explained on pages 28. In addition, it can be used in a Koki ho type healing process in which the violet breath is used to send healing energy into a location in the person's aura or physical body to heal an organ, illness or condition. To use this symbol for healing, draw it on the palms of your hands or visualize it in your mind or draw it in the air in front of you or on the client's body where healing is needed.

Tibetan Fire Serpent

This symbol is also used in the attunement process and is drawn down the back of the student. Doing this causes all the chakras to join together thus allowing the attunement energies to enter the person's energy system more easily. It can also be used in this same way for sessions. Before starting a Reiki treatment, draw the Tibetan Fire Serpent in the air over the front of the client's body with the arch over the crown and then coiling at the root chakra. This will join all the chakras together thus allowing the Reiki energies to flow more evenly throughout the client's system. This symbol can also be used as a regular treatment symbol. Draw it on your palms before placing them on the person. This is a powerful healing symbol and clients often report feeling the energy undulating through them. This undulating action seems to be able to clear blocks more easily and travel more deeply into the energy system. It can also provide a much stronger sensation of heat.

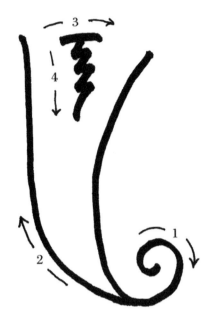

Lightning bolt
has 7 lines

Tibetan
Dai Ko Mio

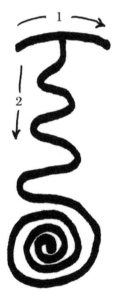

Seven turns including
coil and turn to right of
coil. Coil has 3 turns

Tibetan Fire Serpent

ANTAHKARANA
Ancient Symbol of Healing

Alice Bailey and several other authors of Tibetan philosophy have knowledge of the Antahkarana; you can find this information in a number of books. They describe the Antahkarana as a part of the spiritual anatomy. It is the connection between the physical brain and the Higher Self. It is this connection that must heal and develop if we are to grow spiritually. The Antahkarana symbol depicted and described here represents this connection and activates the Antahkarana whenever you are in its presence.

The science of Radionics indicates that lines drawn on paper create a psychic effect on the space surrounding the drawing and will influence the human aura and chakras in various ways depending on the pattern created. This validates the age-old practice of yantra meditation, which makes use of visual images to purify and evolve the consciousness.

The Antahkarana is an example of this. It is an ancient healing and meditation symbol that has been used in Tibet and China for thousands of years. It is a powerful symbol and simply by having it in your presence, it will create a positive effect on the chakras and aura. When doing healing work, it focuses and deepens the actions of the healing energies involved. It will also neutralize negative energy that has collected in objects such as jewelry or crystals simply by placing the object between two symbols. In addition, it will enhance all healing work including, for example, Reiki, Mahikari, Jin Shin, Polarity Therapy, Chiropractic, Hypnotherapy, and Past

Life Regression. These positive effects have been confirmed over and over by the improved results noted by those using the symbol and by clairvoyant observation by those trained in sensing changes in the aura and chakras.

This symbol is multidimensional. From one perspective it appears to be two dimensional, being made-up of three sevens on a flat surface. The three sevens represent the seven chakras, the seven colors and the seven tones of the musical scale. These three sevens are mentioned in the Book of Revelations as the seven candle sticks, the seven trumpets and the seven seals.

From another perspective this symbol appears as a three dimensional cube. Its energy moves up from two to three dimensions that can be seen and continues up through unseen dimensions all the way to the highest dimension—the dimension of the Higher Self. Historically, the use of this symbol can be traced back through a number of Reiki Masters to an ancient Tibetan meditation technique. The few Tibetan meditation masters who knew of the symbol tended to keep it to themselves, so that the increased value it created for their work would add to their status. For this reason its use has not been widely known.

The Tibetan meditation practice that used the Antahkarana took place in a room lit with candles. In the middle of the room was a large earthenware vessel shaped in an oval, which symbolized the cosmic egg of the universe. The vessel was filled with several inches of water and in the middle was a stool. On the seat of the stool, inlaid in silver, was the Antahkarana Symbol. One wall was covered with copper that was polished to a mirror finish. Tapestries displaying meditation symbols were hung on the opposite wall. A Tibetan Lama meditator would sit on the stool and gaze steadily at the image of the meditation symbol reflected in the polished copper mirror. This yantra meditation would create one-pointedness in the mind of the meditator, uniting the consciousness with the transcendental energies of the meditation symbol while the Antahkarana symbol on the stool would focus the energies generated and cause them to evenly flow through all the chakras.

Directions For Use

The Antahkarana is a special symbol that has its own consciousness. It works directly with your aura and chakras and varies its healing effect depending on what you need at the time of use. Since it is directed by the Higher Self, it always has a beneficial effect and can never be misused or used to cause harm. The symbols can be placed under a Reiki/massage table, or under the bottom of a chair. They can also be placed on the wall or they can be held against your body with the print facing the area that needs healing.

Using the Antahkarana for Meditation

You can meditate directly on the Antahkarana by gazing steadily at it with your eyes relaxed, gently brushing away any thoughts that may come up. With continued practice the image may begin to shift and change or to fade in and out, or it may disappear completely.

This is good because it indicates you have entered a deeper level of meditation and are receiving greater benefit, so do not allow this to disturb you. Continue your steady, relaxed gaze. You may even begin to see pictures in front of the image that are very pleasant and relaxing. A single meditation with the symbol will be beneficial during times of stress; however regular use is best, setting aside 10 to 30 minutes each day for meditation on the Antahkarana. The value you receive will develop along with your mental clarity, and a sense of peace and security will stay with you throughout the day.

There are several variations of the symbol. The large single symbol is more Yin and creates its healing in a gentle way. The smaller single symbol is more Yang and more direct, focused and penetrating. Use your intuition in deciding which one to use.

Multiple Symbols

The Sacred Cross is made of seven symbols crossing each other. This represents the seven major chakras. This symbol will purify your energy and can be used to open the heart. It also attracts Illumined Beings who will bless you and help you with your healing and the healing of others. The square, multiple image symbol made of sixteen symbols will break up blocked and congested energy, and get stuck energy moving. This symbol can also scatter your energy so it is recommended that you follow its use with the single male symbol to create centering and grounding.

If you would like to experiment with these symbols, feel free to make copies of them. For durability you may want to glue them to a cardboard backing, laminate them or place them between two pieces of clear plastic. We also have the symbols on fabric that are more durable and can be draped over one's self or a client during a Reiki session.

The universe is filled with wonder and mystery and as we trust only in the light and boldly explore our true nature, untold value will be revealed to us. The Antahkarana is a symbol that gives freely to all. May you benefit greatly as you explore its use in your journey back to Light.

Please note: you have permission to make as many copies of the symbols as you like for your own use. However, you do not have permission to make copies of the text. Please do not make copies of the text on the Antahkarana or any other part of this manual. Students who are teaching classes can order the manuals directly from www.reikiwebstore.com for use in your classes.

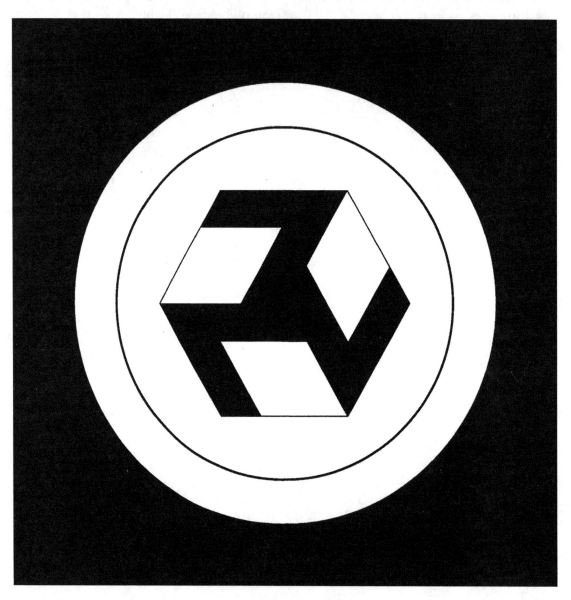

Yang

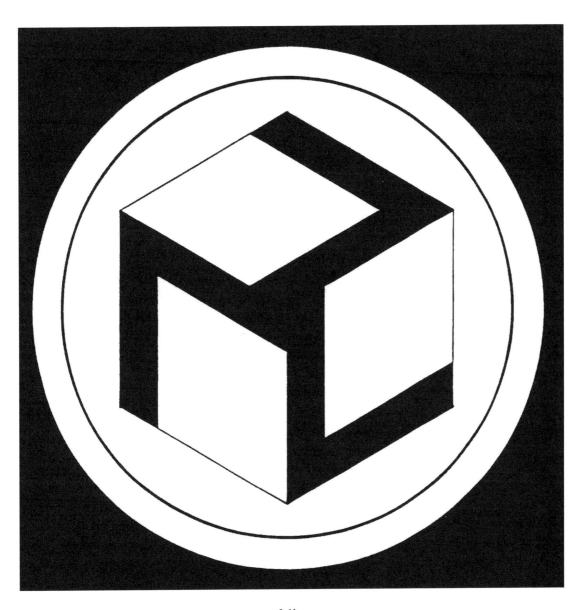

Yin

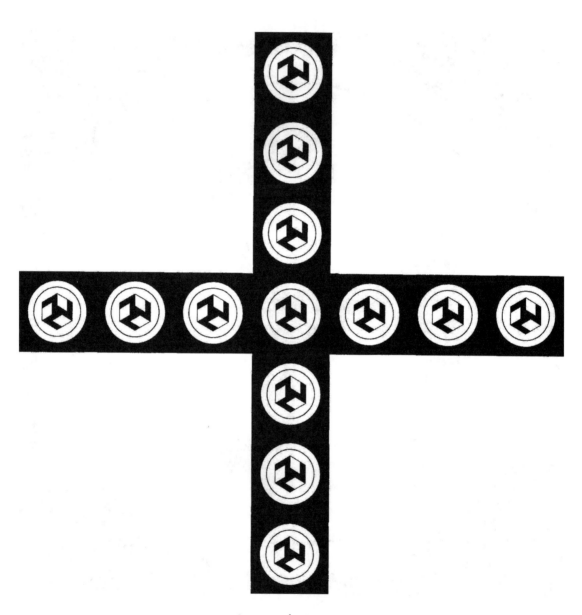

Sacred Cross

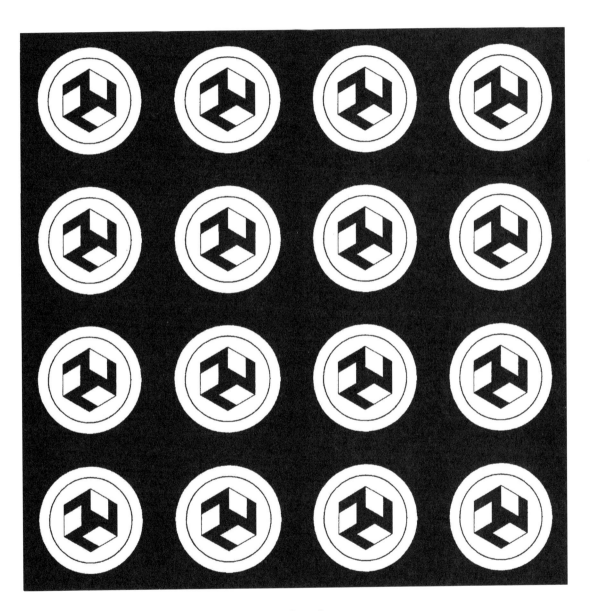

Multiple

Notes

Notes

Attunements

Reiki Attunements

The Reiki attunement is a sacred spiritual initiation that connects the initiate with higher levels of consciousness and an unlimited source of healing energy. It heals and conditions the crown, heart, and palm chakras for their use in channeling Reiki and makes other necessary adjustments in the student's energy system on an individual basis. Reiki is a gift that comes directly from the highest spiritual source and as such should be treated with the greatest respect. It is unique in that there are no requirements necessary in order for it to work and in order for a person to receive the attunements. All that is necessary is for the student to want to receive the attunement and for the teacher to carry out the steps for the attunement. This includes the Reiki Master attunement wherein one can go on to become a Reiki Master/Teacher. Therefore the term "Master" in connection with Reiki is a special one and does not carry with it the same meaning as a spiritual master who is free of all karma, completely purified and fully illuminated. In fact, as stated earlier, the Japanese word for this level is Shinpiden, which means mystery teaching.

Anyone, regardless of the degree of their spiritual development can receive the ability to pass on Reiki to others. Because of this, the level of spiritual development may vary from student to student, but all have the ability to heal. Therefore, all Reiki Master/Teachers are equal in that they all have the ability to pass on Reiki to others. However, their ability as teachers and their understanding of Reiki does vary and is determined mainly by the standards of the individual teacher or school where they have studied, along with personally developed skills and experience.

If it were necessary for a person to be completely pure and free of fault in order to teach Reiki, we would have very few Reiki teachers on this planet. This is the unique value of Reiki; anyone can receive the ability and in a matter of a year or so of dedicated practice become a qualified teacher. This makes Reiki a healing technique of special importance for the period of development in which we presently find ourselves when the consciousness of the planet is advancing so quickly and there is a significantly increased need for spiritual healing.

Giving Reiki Attunements

There are many different techniques in use for giving Reiki attunements. All of them are effective. The process taught by The Center has been distilled from three slightly different techniques and includes the use of two Tibetan symbols as well as the four Usui symbols. Experimentation with emphasis on results was used to develop this attunement process. It is a powerful, yet simple, technique.

Intention is most important in giving the attunements. The Illumined Reiki Spirit Guides who work with you get their cue as to which energies to use and what to do from your intention. This is why you should include a statement in the beginning prayer as to which attunement you intend to use.

This also means that even if you are unable to visualize clearly or not at all, or if you don't draw the symbols perfectly, or if you don't feel anything happening, or if your confidence is low, it doesn't matter. The attunement energies come from a place beyond your personal energy and beyond your ego. Because of this, the attunement will take place anyway simply because of your intention. Attunements work in the same way that Reiki healing energies do. They flow automatically whenever you intend them to.

The first time I did an attunement, it felt as though I was just going through the motions. I couldn't feel anything happening. This lowered my confidence to the point that while doing the attunements I believed that the attunement wasn't working and that I would have to apologize and refund each person's money. I thought I would have to go back to my teacher and find out why it didn't work and be re-attuned. However, I was surprised and pleased afterward when people commented on how powerful the attunement was and how clearly they could feel the new Reiki energies flowing. Some of these students were professional healers and clairvoyants who worked with psychic energies everyday, which qualified them to give an accurate appraisal of the value of a Reiki attunement. From this experience I was impressed with the fact that Reiki attunements work automatically and are not dependent on the energetic state of the person doing the attunements.

How to Give a Reiki Attunement

Before starting the attunement process, ask your students to sit in a row or a circle in straight back chairs. Make sure there is enough room in front and in back for you to walk. Explain about the hands being in the prayer position to start

and that at one point in the attunement process you'll be reaching over and bringing the students hands up onto the top of their head, working with them in that position and then moving them back down in front of them. Demonstrate this so everyone understands. Also explain that you will be placing your hands on the top of the head. (Sometimes during an attunement, a person will get confused and bring the hands up when you place your hands on the top of the head instead of when you touch the left shoulder. If this happens, gently motion their hands back down.) Next guide them into a meditation, grounding them to the earth and connecting them to the spiritual energy above.

Four Parts

While the attunement process is an individual experience and unique adjustments and healing of the student's energy field do take place, generally speaking it seems that the four parts of the attunement process each have a different purpose and cause different things to happen. Part One opens the crown chakra of the student and brings the energies down into your aura and into the aura of the student. In Part Two, the energies enter the hands, the body and chakras of the student. In Part Three, the process is completed by sealing in the attunement, disconnecting the student from the teacher, and permanently connecting the student to the Reiki source. Part Four is a blessing for the students.

Note: If you have any problem visualizing, simply do the best that you can and imagine that the symbols are where you want them to be. It will work just fine and be just as powerful as if you were visualizing them perfectly. It is your intention that is important. Keep in mind that there are powerful Illumined Reiki Guides who will be working with you. In fact, one way to look at it is that they are doing the attunement and you are simply acting as a channel, which is a similar process as when you are giving a Reiki session.

Technique for Each Attunement

As stated, your intention is the most important part of the attunement process so make sure that you state in your mind which attunement you are about to do before you begin, and then simply follow the directions carefully.

It is what goes into the hands that make the difference between the Reiki attunements. This includes when the hands are on top of the head as well as when they are open in front of the heart. Because nothing goes into the hands in the Healing Attunement, the client is not initiated into Reiki and instead the energies are used for healing. In the Reiki I Attunement, only Choku Rei goes into the hands. Note that Choku Rei is used in Reiki I only to empower the hands and the student does not receive the ability to use Choku Rei. In the Reiki II Attunement, the three Reiki II symbols go into the hands and the student is empowered to use them. In the ART attunement, the four Usui symbols go into the hands including the Usui Dai Ko Myo. In the Master attunement, the two Tibetan symbols and the four Usui symbols go into the hands.

Reiki Master Attunement Exercise
Contracting the Hui Yin

A muscular contraction of the Hui Yin (pronounced way yin) point is a necessary part of giving Reiki attunements. The Hui Yin point is between the anus and the genitals. When giving attunements, a special type of high frequency Ki enters your system and passes through the Hui Yin point as part of the process. This point must be held for the entire time you are giving attunements to prevent Ki from escaping from this point. Therefore, it is important to practice holding this point to build up your coordination and muscular strength in this area.

Practice contracting the muscles in this area twenty times in a row and then holding them as long as you can; also practice contracting these muscles continuously while you go about your daily activities.

As you continue, it will become easier and easier and you will be able to contract them for longer periods of time. Also your muscular coordination will develop so that you will be able to isolate the different muscle groups into back, middle and front. It is the middle area that is important to hold for the attunements. You will also develop the ability to very gradually contract the muscles and also to contract them very slightly. It is the development of the ability to contract the Hui Yin point very slightly that will allow you to hold this point for extended periods of time. Practice is the key to success at this exercise.

This exercise is similar to the Kegel birth exercises for woman. Strengthening these muscles is also healthy for a number of other reasons.

Preparations before Beginning an Attunement

Before actually beginning the attunement, follow these steps:

1. Briefly explain the attunement process to your student(s) and especially that you will be touching their head, shoulders, hands, etc. Also, have students place their hands in the Gassho position and lead them in a centering/grounding meditation.

2. Move behind the student and pray out loud or to yourself, asking for the help of your Illumined Reiki Guides and the Illumined Angels and Archangels.

3. Then silently state to yourself and to them which attunement this will be, i.e. Healing Attunement, Reiki I Attunement, etc.

4. Draw a Choku Rei on each wall, the ceiling and the floor.

5. Draw the Tibetan Dai Ko Mio, Usui Dai Ko Myo and Choku Rei on your palm chakras. Draw a large Choku Rei down the front of your body. Then draw Choku Reis on each of your chakras starting with the root chakra and ending with the crown chakra.

6. Draw out all six Reiki symbols in the air in the center of the room intending that their energy fill the room. Then proceed.

The Violet Breath

The Violet Breath is used to place the Tibetan Dai Ko Mio into the heart chakra for the Healing Attunement or into the base of the skull for initiations. It is the use of the Violet Breath and the use of the Master Symbol that begins the attunement process.

1. Contract the Hui Yin point and place your tongue on roof of your mouth.

2. Draw in a breath, imagining it as a column of white light about 1" in diameter coming down through your crown chakra, through your tongue, down the front of the your body (Functional channel) through the Hui Yin point and up the spine (Governing channel) to the center of your head. Imagine the white light filling your head.

3. Imagine the white light as a mist that begins to turn in a clockwise direction as seen from the back of your head. As it rotates see it turn from white to blue to violet so that you have a cloud of violet mist rotating clockwise in your head.

4. Within the violet light picture the Tibetan Dai Ko Mio, which does not rotate.

5. Breathe the Tibetan Dai Ko Mio and violet light into the student's crown chakra.

72

The Violet Breath

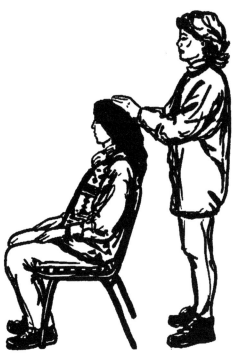

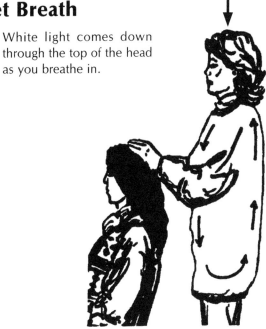

White light comes down through the top of the head as you breathe in.

1. Place your hands on top of the student's head, meditating briefly to gain a rapport.

2. Place your tongue on the roof of your mouth and gently hold the Hui Yin point. Breathe in, imagining white light coming down through the top of your head and flowing down the front of your body, through the Hui Yin point, then up your spine into your head. Imagine your head filling with white light.

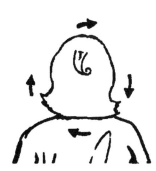

View from the back of your head

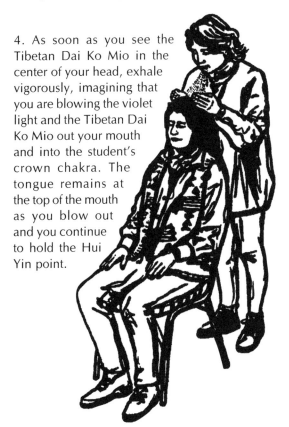

4. As soon as you see the Tibetan Dai Ko Mio in the center of your head, exhale vigorously, imagining that you are blowing the violet light and the Tibetan Dai Ko Mio out your mouth and into the student's crown chakra. The tongue remains at the top of the mouth as you blow out and you continue to hold the Hui Yin point.

3. After your head is filled with white light and while holding the breath, imagine the white light beginning to rotate in a clockwise direction as viewed from the back of your head (moving up on the left side and down on the right). As it rotates, imagine it changing quickly from white to blue to violet. Then imagine the Tibetan Dai Ko Mio in the center of your head. The Tibetan Dai Ko Mio does not rotate.

Reiki Healing Attunement
Explained

A Reiki attunement can be given for healing purposes only. This attunement brings in high frequency healing energies that are more powerful and effective than those given during a regular Reiki treatment. If done before Aura Clearing and a regular Reiki treatment, it will make the treatment more effective by opening the aura and creating a more receptive state. The healing attunement also creates the opportunity for the client's spiritual healers to work with her or him in a more powerful way. This attunement does not initiate the client into Reiki and can be done on anyone. It can be done on more than one client at a time. It must be done in private with no one watching and with the clients eyes closed.

One of the reasons the healing attunement does not initiate the client into Reiki is that the symbols are not placed into the hands.

The most powerful results are achieved by doing a healing attunement first, followed by Aura Clearing as outlined in the Tools & Techniques section and then a standard Reiki treatment using all the hand positions.

Removing Negative Energy

The Reiki healing attunement is highly effective in removing negative energies from the client. It will remove negative energy in the physical body, aura and chakras and work to help release any blocks the client chooses.

Before beginning the healing attunement, explain to the client that she must be willing to let go of the block and any other conditions in her life that the block may have created. She must be willing to make important changes in attitude about herself and her life concerning the issues involved and to become aware of those issues in new ways. Have the client focus on the block with the intention of releasing it during the healing attunement.

Empowering Goals

The healing attunement can also be used to empower goals. If there is a goal the client has had trouble achieving, it is likely that there is something that needs to heal before she can achieve it. There may be unconscious, negative feelings and thoughts about the goal that are blocking its achievement such as fear of failure or fear of success. Having the client focus on these blocks will cause them to be released during the Healing Attunement.

During the Healing Attunement, it is also possible to receive insight about the goal and guidance for making plans. Sometimes a particular goal is not in harmony with a person's life path. If this is the case, the client may become aware of this during the healing attunement.

Have the client focus on the goal and be willing to take responsibility for doing whatever is necessary to achieve it while being open to new ideas and attitudes about it. A willingness to release unconscious, negative attitudes about the goal is also necessary.

Preparations for Healing Attunement

Follow these steps first before doing your own preparations. The client should be sitting with her feet flat on the floor and her hands palms down on her legs. The client's eyes should remain closed throughout the healing attunement with her attention focused inwardly on her purpose. A short meditation can be done to connect the person to the positive energies of the earth and to the positive energies from above. It is important for the client to locate the area in which the cause of the problem is located and to define its other qualities. Use the following steps to do this. (These are very similar steps to those used in Aura Clearing located in the Tools & Techniques section.)

Steps

The first step is to give the cause of the problem an identity. This will allow the client and practitioner to focus directly on the cause and release it. Giving the problem an identity can be very healing in itself as it allows one to bring the cause into awareness, where it can be dealt with. This involves finding the location of the block and becoming aware of what it looks like.

1. Ask the client to think about the issue she would like to have healed. Note that it is not necessary for her to tell you what the issue is, just for her to think about it. This confidentiality can be very helpful for many clients as some issues are so sensitive that the client may not want to let anyone know about what the issue is.

2. Ask her to close her eyes and meditate on the issue. Ask the client: "If the original cause of this issue were to be located somewhere in your physical body, where would it be?" This is often easy because the client will feel tension or pain in an area of the body when she thinks of the issue. If she has difficulty choosing an area, just ask the client to guess and assure her that there is no wrong answer. Whichever area she chooses will work.

3. Ask her to imagine that she is looking into the area she has chosen and ask her, "If this issue had a shape, what shape would it have?"

4. Do the same thing to find the color, texture, weight, temperature and sound that the shape makes so that the client has a clear energetic image of the block. Remember that any answer is okay and that the client doesn't have to answer all of the questions.

Healing Attunement

Preparation: Prepare yourself and the room using the steps on pp. 72. Prepare the client using the steps on pp. 75.

Part One
1. **Fire Serpent:** Move behind the client and hold the space with your non-dominant hand by placing it about 8" from the clients head/shoulder area. Draw the Fire Serpent down the back starting with the arch over the top of the head, then undulating down the back and coiling at the base of the spine.
2. **Rapport:** Place both hands on top of the head and close your eyes, meditating briefly to gain energetic rapport with the client.
3. **Violet Breath:** Bring your tongue to the top of your mouth, contract the Hui Yin point and do the Violet Breath. (Remember, you must continue holding the Hui Yin point and continue to keep your tongue touching the top of your mouth throughout the remainder of the attunement.) Open your hands and exhale into the crown chakra picturing the Tibetan Dai Ko Mio (TDKM) moving from the middle of your head, out with your breath and into the client's crown chakra. Then hold the space with your non-dominant hand and motion the TDKM to the heart chakra using your dominant hand in three steps by pointing to the crown chakra, then the center of the head and finally the back of the heart. As you do this say, "Dai Ko Mio" three times in mantra-like fashion, once at each position. (Note, this is a different process than when initiating a person into Reiki. When initiating into Reiki, the symbols go to the base of the brain; when giving a healing attunement, the symbols go to the heart.)
4. **Symbols:** Continue to hold the space and draw the Usui Dai Ko Myo (UDKM) over the head vertically. Then motion the UDKM to the heart chakra in three steps by pointing to the crown chakra, then the center of the head and finally the back of the heart. As you do this say, Dai Ko Myo three times in mantra-like fashion, once at each position.
5. **Repeat** step four with Choku Rei, Sei heki and Hon Sha Ze Sho Nen.

Complete the process with each person and continue to Part Two.

Part Two
1. **Front Symbols:** Move to the front, hold the space and draw the Tibetan Dai Ko Mio over the front part of the crown chakra. Then repeat Dai Ko Mio three times as you guide the symbol through the third eye, the heart and then into the solar plexus. Gently tap the top of the head three times with the fingertips.

     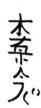

2. **Repeat** the above step with the Usui Dai Ko Myo, Choku Rei, Sei heki and Hon Sha Ze Sho Nen.

3. **Blowing with Hand Motion:** Gently blow toward the solar plexus, and continue blowing as you move up to the heart, the third eye, and the crown. Continue blowing back down to the solar plexus, then back up to the crown. The blowing is done in one smooth, continuous breath so make sure you have enough air in your lungs when you start and that you do not blow out too quickly. Blow up, then down, then back up. As you blow, use your hands with palms facing the direction of motion to guide the energy, placing a strong intention on the last upward motion to sweep out all negative energy and move it up and completely out.

Complete the process with each person and continue to Part Three.

Part Three

1. **Affirmation:** Move behind the client again. Place your hands on the client's shoulders and look down through the crown chakra imagining that you can see into the heart. Look for a soft pink ball of light (could also be white, green, lavender, or gold), or imagine one being there. Lovingly place a positive affirmation in the client's heart and subconscious mind by repeating it to yourself three times, intending that it be accepted by the subconscious mind to enter the heart. Use affirmations such as "You are completely healed by Divine love now" or "You are completely guided and cared for by God now" or "You are empowered by Divine love, wisdom and power to achieve your highest spiritual purpose now."

2. **Sealing:** Place your dominant hand on the back of the client's heart chakra, and the non-dominant hand on the shoulder. Repeat this phrase three times to yourself: "I perfectly seal this healing process with Divine love and wisdom" while picturing a door with Choku Rei on it being closed over the back of the heart chakra. While you do this, intend, will and feel that the healing process is sealed and complete.

3. **Blessing:** Place your hands on the client's shoulders with the feeling that both you and the client have been blessed by the experience.

Part Four

1. **Final Blessing:** Move in front of the client and hold your hands with fingers pointed in toward your heart chakra and the backs of your hands facing each other. Say a prayer asking that the client be deeply blessed and healed.

2. Inhale and hold the breath briefly, then exhale while releasing the Hui Yin point and tongue and intending that the releasing energy act as a blessing for the client. As you release, motion the hands outward toward the client with the intention of bestowing a blessing on her.

3. Ask the client to breath slowly and deeply, and to slowly open her eyes.

4. Ask the client "What does the shape look like now?" If the shape is gone, then the healing is complete. If all or part of the shape is still there, more healing is needed. Use Aura Clearing to remove any part of the shape that is still left.

Healing Attunement
Quick Guide

Preparation: Work with the client to explain the process and to determine the location, the shape, color etc. of the issue, pp. 78. Prepare yourself and the room using the steps on pp. 72.

Part One
1. **Fire Serpent**

2. **Rapport:** Hands on top of head.

3. **Violet Breath:** pp. 72-73.

4. **Symbols:** Draw them over the crown, then move them into the heart in three steps.

Part Two
1. **Front Symbols:** Draw them over the front of the head and move them into the solar plexus. Remember to tap after each symbol.

2. **Blowing and Hand Motion**

Part Three
1. **Affirmation:** From behind through top of head.

2. **Sealing**

3. **Blessing**

Part Four
1. **Final Blessing**

2. **Bring client back**

3. **Ask about shape:** If more work is needed use Aura Clearing pp. 28.

Reiki I Attunement

Note in the Reiki I attunement, only Choku Rei goes into the hands, both when they are on top of the head and when they are open in front. The use of Choku Rei is only to empower the hands and does not give the student the use of Choku Rei during sessions.

Preparation: Prepare yourself and the room using the steps on pp. 72.

Part One
1. **Fire Serpent:** Move behind the client and hold the space with your non-dominant hand. Draw the Fire Serpent down the back starting with the arch over the top of the head, then undulating down the back and coiling at the base of the spine.
2. **Rapport:** Place both hands on top of the head and close your eyes, meditating briefly to gain energetic rapport with the student.
3. **Violet Breath:** Bring your tongue to the top of your mouth, contract the Hui Yin point and do the Violet Breath. (Remember, you must continue holding the Hui Yin point and continue to keep your tongue touching the top of your mouth throughout all the steps of the attunement.) Open your hands and exhale into the crown chakra, picturing the Tibetan Dai Ko Mio (TDKM) moving from the middle of your head, out with your breath and into the student's crown chakra. Then, while holding the space with your non-dominant hand, motion the TDKM to the base of the skull in three steps by pointing to the crown chakra, then the center of the head and finally the base of the skull. As you do this say "Dai Ko Mio" three times to yourself in mantra-like fashion, once at each position.
4. **Symbols:** Continue to hold the space and draw the Usui Dai Ko Myo (UDKM) over the head vertically. Then motion the UDKM to the base of the skull in three steps by pointing to the crown chakra, then the center of the head and finally the base of the skull. As you do this say Dai Ko Myo three times in mantra-like fashion to yourself, once at each position.
5. **Repeat** step four with Sei heki and Hon Sha Ze Sho Nen. (note that you have temporarily skipped Choku Rei.)
6. **Bring Hands Up:** Reach over and bring the student's prayer clasped hands up to the top of the student's head.
7. **Symbol into Hands:** While holding the students hands with your non-dominant hand, draw Choku Rei in the air over the student's hands. Then motion "Choku Rei" to the base of the skull in three steps by pointing to the hands and crown, then the center of the head and finally the base of the skull. As you do this say, Choku Rei three times in mantra-like fashion to yourself, once at each position.
8. **Return Hands:** Gently move the student's hands from the top of their head, to back down in front of the student's heart.

     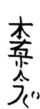

Complete this process with each person, then move in front and proceed with Part Two.

Part Two

1. **Symbol into Hands**: Move in front of the student and open the student's hands flat, then support them with your non-dominate hand under their hands. With your dominant hand, draw Choku Rei in the air above the hands. Picture the symbol moving into the hands as you silently chant the secret name of "Choku Rei" three times and motion the energy in. Pat the hands three times. Note that motioning and patting the hands are separate steps.

2. **Blow on Hands:** Bring the student's hands together and move them back in front of the heart. Hold your hands over his hands, or lightly touch them and blow over the hands, then down to the solar plexus, then up to the third eye and crown, then back over the hands to the solar plexus, and ending at the hands with an extra large puff of air.

Complete the process with each student and continue to Part Three.

Part Three

1. **Affirmation:** Move behind the student and place your hands on the student's shoulders and look down through the crown chakra, imagining that you can see all the way down to the root chakra at the base of the spine. Look for a red ball of light or imagine one being there in the root chakra. Place a positive affirmation there such as "You are a powerful and successful Reiki I practitioner filled with God's love and light" or "Divine love and wisdom guides and empowers you in your use of Reiki." Repeat this three times and imagine you are placing this into the root chakra and intending that it be accepted by the subconscious mind of the student.

2. **Sealing:** Bring your hands together, placing your thumbs at the base of the skull. Repeat this phrase three times to yourself: "I now seal this process with Divine love and wisdom" while picturing a door with Choku Rei on it being closed. While you do this, intend, will and feel that the process is sealed and complete and that the student is now connected directly to the Reiki source.

3. **Blessing:** Place your hands on the student's shoulders while feeling that both of you have been blessed by the experience.

Part Four

1. **Final Blessing:** Move in front of the student and hold your hands with fingers pointed in toward your heart chakra and the backs of your hands facing each other. Say a prayer asking that the student be deeply blessed and healed.

2. Inhale and hold the breath briefly, then exhale while releasing the Hui Yin point and tongue and intending that the releasing energy act as a blessing for the student. As you release, motion the hands outward toward the student with the intention of bestowing a blessing on him.

3. Ask the student to breath slowly and deeply, and to slowly open his eyes. Then either place the student's hands over his heart or ask the student to do so and ask him to meditate on Reiki.

Reiki I Attunement
Quick Guide

Preparation: Prepare yourself and the room using the steps on pp. 72.

Part One

1. **Fire Serpent**

2. **Rapport:** Hands on top of head.

3. **Violet Breath:** pp. 72-73.

4. **Symbols:** Draw the UDKM over crown, then move it into the base of the skull in three steps. Do the same with the other symbols, remembering to temporarily skip the Choku Rei, then add it as last step after bringing the students hands over the top of their head.

Part Two

1. **Front. Symbol into Hands:** Open hands and draw the Choku Rei over the hands, motion it in, then gently tap three times.

2. **Blowing on Hands:** Down, up, down, up while holding hands.

Part Three

1. **Behind. Affirmation:** From behind through top of head, into root chakra.

2. **Sealing:** Thumbs to base of skull.

3. **Blessing:** Both you and student are blessed.

Part Four

1. **Final Blessing**

2. **Bring student back:** Student places hands over heart and meditates on Reiki.

Reiki II Attunement

Preparation: Prepare yourself and the room using the steps on pp. 72.

Part One

Note that when giving the Reiki II Attunement, you will be placing the three Reiki II symbols in the hands, both when they are on top of the head and when they are held out in front.

1. **Fire Serpent:** Move behind the client and hold the space with your non-dominant hand. Draw the Fire Serpent down the back starting with the arch over the top of the head, then undulating down the back and coiling at the base of the spine.

2. **Rapport:** Place both hands on top of the head and close your eyes, meditating briefly to gain energetic rapport with the student.

3. **Violet Breath:** Place your tongue on the roof of your mouth, contract the Hui Yin point and do the Violet Breath. (Remember, you must continue holding the Hui Yin point and continue to keep your tongue touching the top of your mouth throughout all the steps of the attunement.) Open your hands and exhale into the crown chakra picturing the Tibetan Dai Ko Mio (TDKM) moving from the middle of your head, out with your breath and into the student's crown chakra. Then motion the TDKM to the base of the skull in three steps by pointing to the crown chakra, then the center of the head and finally the base of the skull. As you do this say, "Dai Ko Mio" three times in mantra-like fashion to yourself, once at each position.

4. **Symbols:** Continue to hold the space with your non-dominant hand and draw the Usui Dai Ko Myo (UDKM) over the head vertically. Then motion the UDKM to the base of the skull in three steps by pointing to the crown chakra, then the center of the head and finally the base of the skull. As you do this say, "Dai Ko Myo" three times in mantra-like fashion to yourself, once at each position.

5. **Bring Hands Up:** Reach over and bring the student's prayer clasped hands up to the top of the student's head.

6. **Symbols into Hands**: Hold the students hands with your non-dominant hand and draw Choku Rei in the air over the hands. Then motion Choku Rei to the base of the skull in three steps by pointing to the hands and crown, then the center of the head and finally the base of the skull. As you do this say Choku Rei three times to yourself in mantra-like fashion, once at each position. Do the same with Sei heki and Hon Sha Ze Sho Nen.

7. **Return Hands:** Gently move the student's hands from the top of his head, back down to in front of the student's heart.

     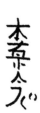

Complete this process with each person, then move to the front and proceed with Part Two.

Part Two

1. **Symbols into Hands:** Move to the front, and open the student's hands flat then support them with your non-dominant hand under his hands. With your dominant hand, draw Choku Rei in the air above the hands. Picture the symbol moving into the hands as you silently chant "Choku Rei" three times and motion the energy in. Pat the hands three times. Do the same with Sei heki and Hon Sha Ze Sho Nen. Note that motioning and patting the hands are separate steps.

2. **Blow on Hands:** Bring the student's hands together and move them back in front of his heart. Hold your hands over his hands or lightly touch them and blow over the hands, then down to the solar plexus, up to the third eye and crown, back over the hands to the solar plexus, and ending at the hands with a larger puff of air at the end.

Complete the process with each student and continue to Part Three.

Part Three

1. **Affirmation:** Move behind the student and place your hands on the student's shoulders and look down through the crown chakra, imagining that you can see all the way down to the root chakra at the base of the spine. Look for a red ball of light or imagine one being there in the root chakra. Place a positive affirmation there such as "You are a powerful and successful Reiki II practitioner, filled with God's love and wisdom." Repeat this three times and imagine you are placing this into the root chakra and intending that it be accepted by the subconscious mind of the student.

2. **Sealing:** Bring your hands together, placing your thumbs at the base of the skull. Repeat this phrase three times to yourself: "I now seal this process with Divine love and wisdom," while picturing a door with Choku Rei on it being closed. While you do this, intend, will and feel that the process is sealed and complete and that the student is now connected directly to the Reiki source.

3. **Blessing:** Place your hands on the student's shoulders while feeling that both of you have been blessed by the experience.

Part Four

1. **Final Blessing:** Move in front of the student and hold your hands with fingers pointed in toward your heart chakra with the backs of your hands facing each other. Silently say a prayer asking that the student(s) be deeply blessed and healed.

2. Inhale and hold the breath briefly, then exhale while releasing the Hui Yin point and tongue and intending that the releasing energy act as a blessing for the student. As you release, motion the hands outward toward the student with the intention of bestowing a blessing on him.

3. Ask the student to breathe slowly and deeply, and to slowly open his eyes. Then either place the student's hands over his heart or ask the student(s) to do so and ask the student to meditate on the Reiki II symbols.

Reiki II Attunement
Quick Guide

Preparation: Prepare yourself and the room using the steps on pp. 72.

Part One – Behind
1. **Fire Serpent**

2. **Rapport:** Hands on top of head.

3. **Violet Breath:** pp. 72-73.

4. **Symbols:** Draw the UDKM over crown, then move it into the base of the skull in three steps. Bring hands up and do same with the three Reiki II symbols. Return hands.

Part Two – Front
1. **Symbol into Hands:** Open hands and draw the three Reiki II symbols over the hands, motion each in, then gently tap three times.

2. Blow on Hands: Down, up, down, up while holding hands.

Part Three – Behind
1. **Affirmation:** From behind through top of head into root chakra.

2. **Sealing:** Thumbs to base of skull.

3. **Blessing:** Both you and student are blessed.

Part Four – Front
1. **Final Blessing**

2. **Bring student back:** Ask student to place hands over heart and meditate on the Reiki II symbols.

Notes

Advanced Reiki Training Attunement

Preparation: Prepare yourself and the room using the steps on pp. 72.

The difference between the Reiki II Attunement and the ART Attunement is what goes into the hands. In ART the Usui Dai Ko Myo, along with the other three symbols, are placed in the hands, both when they are on the top of the head in Part One, as well as in Part Two when they are held flat in front of the heart.

Part One

1. **Fire Serpent:** Move behind the client and hold the space with your non-dominant hand. Draw the Fire Serpent down the back starting with the arch over the top of the head, then undulating down the back and coiling at the base of the spine.
2. **Rapport:** Place both hands on top of the head and close your eyes, meditating briefly to gain energetic rapport with the student.
3. **Violet Breath:** Place your tongue on the roof of your mouth, contract the Hui Yin point and do the Violet Breath. (Remember, you must continue holding the Hui Yin point and continue to keep your tongue touching the top of your mouth throughout all the steps of the attunement.) Open your hands and exhale into the crown chakra picturing the Tibetan Dai Ko Mio (TDKM) moving from the middle of your head, out with your breath and into the student's crown chakra. Then motion the TDKM to the base of the skull in three steps by pointing to the crown chakra, then the center of the head and finally the base of the skull. As you do this, say "Dai Ko Mio" three times in mantra-like fashion to yourself, once at each position.
4. **Bring Hands Up:** Reach over and bring the student's prayer clasped hands up to the top of the student's head.
5. **Symbols:** Continue to hold the space and draw the Usui Dai Ko Myo (UDKM) over the hands vertically. Then motion the UDKM to the base of the skull in three steps by pointing to the hands and crown chakra, then the center of the head and finally the base of the skull. As you do this say, "Dai Ko Mio" three times in mantra-like fashion to yourself, once at each position. Repeat this step with Choku Rei, Sei heki and Hon Sha Ze Sho Nen.
6. **Return Hands:** Gently move the student's hands from the top of his head, back down to in front of the heart.

Complete this process with each person, then move to the front and proceed with Part Two.

    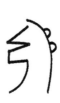 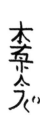

Part Two

1. **Symbols into Hands:** Move to the front and open the student's hands flat, then support them with your non-dominant hand placed under their hands. With your dominant hand draw the Usui Dai Ko Myo in the air above the hands. Picture the symbol moving into the hands as you silently chant the secret name of the Usui Dai Ko Myo three times and motion the energy in. Pat the hands three times. Do the same with Choku Rei, Sei heki and Hon Sha Ze Sho Nen. Note that motioning and patting the hands are separate steps.
2. **Blow on Hands:** Bring the student's hands together and move them back in front of his heart. Hold your hands over his hands or lightly touch them and blow over the hands, down to the solar plexus, up to the third eye and crown, back over the hands to the solar plexus, and ending at the hands with a larger puff at the end.

Complete the process with each student and continue to Part Three.

Part Three

1. **Affirmation:** Move behind the student and place your hands on the student's shoulders and look down through the crown chakra, imagining that you can see all the way down to the root chakra at the base of the spine. Look for a red ball of light or imagine one being there in the root chakra. Place a positive affirmation there such as "You are a powerful and successful Advanced Reiki Practitioner filled with God's love and wisdom." Repeat this three times and imagine you are placing this into the root chakra and intending that it be accepted by the subconscious mind of the student.
2. **Sealing:** Bring your hands together, placing your thumbs at the base of the skull. Repeat this phrase three times to yourself: "I now seal this process with Divine love and wisdom" while picturing a door with Choku Rei on it being closed and locked. While you do this, intend, will and feel that the process is sealed and complete and that the student is now connected directly to the Reiki source.
3. **Blessing:** Place your hands on the student's shoulders, while feeling that both of you have been blessed by the experience.

Part Four

1. **Final Blessing:** Move to the front of the student(s) and hold your hands with fingers pointed in toward your heart chakra and the backs of your hands facing each other. Silently say a prayer asking that the student(s) be deeply blessed and healed.
2. Inhale and hold the breathe briefly, then exhale while releasing the Hui Yin point and tongue and intending that the releasing energy act as a blessing for the student(s). As you release, motion the hands outward toward the student(s) with the intention of bestowing a blessing on them.
3. Ask the student(s) to breath slowly and deeply, and to slowly open his/their eyes. Then either place the student's hands over his heart or ask the student(s) to do so and to meditate on the Usui Dai Ko Myo.

ART Attunement
Quick Guide

Preparation: Prepare yourself and the room using the steps on pp. 72.

Part One – Behind
1. **Fire Serpent**

2. **Rapport:** Hands on top of head.

3. **Violet Breath:** pp. 72-73.

4. **Symbols:** Bring hands up after violet breath. Draw UDKM and three Reiki II symbols over hands, then direct them to crown, center of head and base of skull.

Part Two – Front
1. **Symbol into Hands:** Open hands and draw the UDKM and the three Reiki II symbols over the hands, motion each in as you say its name three times, then gently tap three times.

2. **Blow on Hands:** Down, up, down, up while holding hands.

Part Three – Behind
1. **Affirmation:** From behind through top of head, into root chakra.

2. **Sealing:** Thumbs to base of skull.

3. **Blessing:** Both you and student are blessed.

Part Four – Front
1. **Final Blessing**

2. **Bring client back:** Then ask student to place hands over heart and meditate on the UDKM symbol.

Reiki Master Attunement

Preparation: Prepare yourself and the room using the steps on pp. 72.

In the Reiki Master Attunement you will be placing all six symbols into the hands, both when they are on top of the head and when they are open in front of the heart. This includes doing the Violet Breath into the hands when they are on top of the head. The Reiki Master Attunement gives the student the ability to give Reiki attunements.

Part One
1. **Fire Serpent:** Move behind the client and hold the space with your non-dominant hand. Draw the Fire Serpent down the back starting with the arch over the top of the head, then undulating down the back and coiling at the base of the spine.
2. **Rapport:** Place both hands on top of the head and close your eyes, meditating briefly to gain energetic rapport with the client.
3. **Bring Hands Up:** Reach over and bring the student's prayer clasped hands up to the top of the student's head.
3. **Violet Breath**: Place your tongue on the top of your mouth and contract the Hui Yin point. **Then do the Violet Breath through the hands** by holding the hands with both of your hands, then opening your hands slightly when blowing the Violet Breath into them. (Remember, you must continue holding the Hui Yin point and continue to keep your tongue touching the top of your mouth during all the steps of the attunement.) As you do the Violet Breath, picture the Tibetan Dai Ko Mio (TDKM) moving from the middle of your head, out with your breath, through the student's hands and into the crown chakra. Then motion the TDKM to the base of the skull in three steps by pointing to the hands and crown chakra, then the center of the head and finally the base of the skull. As you do this say, "Dai Ko Mio" three times in mantra-like fashion to yourself, once at each position.
5. **Symbols:** Continue to hold the space and draw the Fire Serpent over the hands vertically. Then motion it to the base of the skull in three steps by pointing to the hands and crown chakra, then the center of the head and finally the base of the skull. As you do this say, "Fire Serpent" three times in mantra-like fashion to yourself, once at each position. Repeat this step with the Usui Dai Ko Myo, Choku Rei, Sei heki and Hon Sha Ze Sho Nen.
6. **Return Hands:** Gently move the student's hands from the top of her head, back down to in front of her heart.

Complete this process with each person, then move to the front and proceed with Part Two.

     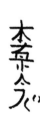

Part Two

1. **Symbols into Hands:** Move to the front and open the student's hands flat, then support them with your non-dominant hand under their hands. With your dominant hand, draw the Tibetan Dai Ko Mio in the air above the hands. Picture the symbol moving into the hands as you silently chant "Dai Ko Mio" three times and motion the energy in. Pat the hands three times. Do the same with the Fire Serpent, Usui Dai Ko Myo, Choku Rei, Sei heki and Hon Sha Ze Sho Nen. Note that motioning and patting the hands are separate steps.
2. **Blow on Hands:** Bring the student's hands together and move them back in front of her heart. Hold your hands over her hands and blow over the hands, down to the solar plexus, up to the third eye and crown, back over the hands to the solar plexus, and ending at the hands.

Complete the process with each student and continue on to Part Three.

Part Three

1. **Affirmation:** Move behind the student and place your hands on the student's shoulders and look down through the crown chakra, imagining that you can see all the way down to the root chakra at the base of the spine. Look for a red ball of light or imagine one being there in the root chakra. Place a positive affirmation there such as "You are a powerful and successful Reiki Master filled with God's love and light." Repeat this three times and imagine you are placing this into the root chakra and intending that it be accepted by the subconscious mind of the student.
2. **Sealing:** Bring your hands together, placing your thumbs at the base of the skull. Repeat this phrase three times to yourself: "I now seal this process with Divine love and wisdom" while picturing a door with Choku Rei on it being closed and locked. While you do this, intend, will and feel that the process is sealed and complete and that the student is now connected directly to the Reiki source.
3. **Blessing:** Place your hands on the student's shoulders while feeling that both of you have been blessed by the experience.

Part Four

1. **Final Blessing:** Move to the front of the student and hold your hands with fingers pointed in toward your heart chakra with the backs of your hands facing each other. Silently say a prayer asking that the student(s) be deeply blessed and healed.
2. Inhale and hold the breath briefly, then exhale while releasing the Hui Yin point and tongue and intending that the releasing energy act as a blessing for the student(s). As you release, motion the hands outward toward the student(s) with the intention of bestowing a blessing on them.
3. Ask the student to breathe slowly and deeply, and to slowly open her eyes. Then either place the student's hands over her heart or ask the student(s) to do so and ask student(s) to meditate on the Tibetan symbols.

Reiki Master Attunement
Quick Guide

Preparation: Prepare yourself and the room using the steps on pp. 72.

Part One – Behind
1. **Fire Serpent**

2. **Rapport:** Hands on top of head.

3. **Violet Breath:** pp. 72-73. This is done through the hands. Then guide the TDKM through the hands, into the crown, center of head and base of skull. Do the same with the TFS, UDKM and the three Reiki II symbols.

Part Two – Front
1. **Symbol into Hands:** Open hands and draw the TDKM, TFS, UDKM and the three Reiki II symbols over the hands, motion each in as you say its name three times, then gently tap three times.

2. **Blow on Hands:** Down, up, down, up while holding hands.

Part Three – Behind
1. **Affirmation:** From behind through top of head, into root chakra.

2. **Sealing:** Thumbs to base of skull.

3. **Blessing:** Both you and student are blessed.

Part Four – Front
1. **Final Blessing**

2. **Bring student back:** Then ask student to place hands over heart and meditate on the TDKM and Fire Serpent.

Notes

Attuning Yourself

There are several ways you can give yourself an attunement. One involves using a Teddy Bear. Place the Teddy Bear in a chair and draw the Hon Sha Ze Sho Nen symbol down the front. Then say, the symbol name three times and say "As I give an attunement to this teddy bear, I give an attunement to myself." Then perform the full attunement process on the teddy bear, and you will receive the attunement.

Another way is to sit in a chair meditating for a moment, then do your preparations for the attunement you intend to give yourself. Next stand up, but as you stand up imagine you are leaving your astral body in the chair. Move around to the back and imagine you are still seated in the chair and begin the attunement by drawing the fire serpent down the back and doing the violet breath. Proceed with all the steps of the attunement imagining you are actually seated in the chair. When you are done sit down on the chair imagining as you do so that you are moving back into your astral body. As you sit there place your hands on your heart and meditate on the attunement energy you have just received. Some use this method to give themselves the Master attunement every day for a month with amazing results!

Distant Attunement

It is possible to send a Healing Attunement to others at a distance. Use a Teddy Bear or a pillow placed in a chair to represent the person to whom you intend to send the Healing Attunement. You can call the person on the phone and ask the person to be seated in a chair. Then go through the preparations on the phone including finding the location, shape, color etc. of the issue. Ask the person to close her/his eyes and focus on the shape and be willing to let it go. Then put the phone down and draw Hon Sha Ze Sho Nen over the Teddy Bear or pillow and repeat the person's name three times, intending that the Teddy Bear or pillow represents her/him and that the attunement will go to her/him. Then proceed with the attunement process. When you are done, pick up the phone and ask what the shape looks like now. If it is gone you are done, but if some of the shape is still there, proceed with Aura Clearing to remove the last part of the shape. Use the distant attunement process to do the Healing Attunement only. The initiations for Reiki I, II, ART or Master should only be done in person as part of a Reiki class.

Practice Attunements

Practice doing attunements on friends and family. Reiki support groups are a great place to practice attunements. The initiatory attunements should only be practiced on people who already have received the attunement you want to practice. While an attunement will last a lifetime and no additional attunements are necessary in order for the person to continue to have Reiki, additional attunements strengthen and refine the Reiki energy they already have and can also create spiritual experiences. The healing attunements can be done on anyone.

The Western/Takata System of Attunements

This information is sacred. Do not show it to anyone or leave it where others could read it.

The following is an outline of the Western/Takata style of attunements. In this system the Violet Breath, the Tibetan Symbols and holding the tongue and the Hui Yin are not used. There are four attunements for Reiki I, one attunement for Reiki II (although some were taught two attunements for Reiki II) and one attunement for Reiki Master. There is no advanced attunement in the Western/Takata system. The symbols are also placed in the third eye. (You can add this step to your Usui/Tibetan Attunements if you are guided to do so. This is in Part Two, Step 2.)

Begin each attunement process using the instructions on pp. 72. Then proceed with the following:

First Degree Attunement

You will be placing only Choku Rei into the hands (and third eye) during all four attunements for First Degree. This applies when the hands are on the head as well as when they are open in front.

First of Four Attunements

Part One (back)

1. Place both hands on top of the head and close your eyes, meditating briefly to gain energetic rapport with the student.

2. Draw the Usui Dai Ko Myo over the head and while repeating the secret name of the Usui Dai Ko Myo three times to yourself in mantra-like fashion, picture the symbol moving into the crown chakra through the head and lodging in the base of the brain, guiding it with your non-dominant hand.

3. Reach over and move the student's prayer clasped hands to the top of her head.

4. Draw Choku Rei in the air over the hands. Then picture the symbol moving into the hands and down into the crown chakra through the head and lodging in the base of the brain, while silently chanting Choku Rei three times.

5. Gently move the student's hands from the top of their head directing them back down in front of the heart.

Complete the process with each student and proceed to Part Two.

Part Two (front)

1. Move to the front and open the student's hands flat while holding your non-dominant hand under the student's hands.

2. Draw Choku Rei in front of the student's third eye. Chant Choku Rei three times as you picture it moving into the head through the third eye.

3. With your dominant hand draw Choku Rei in the air above the student's hands. Picture the symbol moving into the hands as you silently chant Choku Rei three times and motion the symbol into the student's hands. Pat the hands three times.

4. Bring the student's hands together and move them back to in front of the student's heart. Blow over the hands, up to the third eye and crown, and back over the hands to the solar plexus and back to the hands.

Complete the process with each student then continue to Part Three.

Part Three (back)

1. Place your hands on the student's shoulders and look down through the crown chakra imagining that you can see into the student's heart chakra. Place a positive affirmation such as "You are a successful and confident Reiki healer" or "Divine love and wisdom guides and empowers you in your use of Reiki" into the heart of the student by silently repeating it three times, intending that it be accepted by the subconscious mind of the student.

2. Bring your hands together, placing your thumbs at the base of the skull. Repeat the phrase "I seal this process with Divine love and wisdom" while picturing a door with Choku Rei on it being closed and locked. While you do this, intend, will and feel that the process is sealed and complete and the student is now connected directly to the Reiki Source.

3. Place your palms on the student's shoulders and repeat the affirmation, "We are both blessed by this process" or hold this feeling for several seconds.

4. Move to the front. Ask the student(s) to place their hands palm down on their legs and to breath deeply and slowly while opening their eyes. You may add a final blessing of your own at this point if you choose.

Second and Third of Four Attunements

Note that the second and third attunements for First Degree Reiki are exactly the same.

Part One (back)

1. Place both hands on top of the head and close your eyes, meditating briefly to gain energetic rapport with the student.

2. Draw the Usui Dai Ko Myo above the head while silently repeating "Dai Ko Myo" three times in mantra-like fashion. Picture the symbol moving into the crown chakra through the head and lodging in the base of the brain, guiding it with your right hand.

3. Draw Hon Sha Ze Sho Nen above the head while silently repeating Hon Sha Ze Sho Nen three times in mantra-like fashion. Picture the symbol moving into the crown chakra through the head and lodging in the base of the brain, guiding it with your right hand.

4. Reach over and move the student's prayer clasped hands to the top of their head.

5. Draw Choku Rei in the air above the hands. Then picture the symbol moving into the hands, down into the crown chakra through the head and lodging in the base of the brain, while silently chanting Choku Rei three times.

6. Gently move the student's hands from the top of their head directing them back down to in front of the heart.

Complete the process with each student and continue to Part Two.

Part Two (front)
1. Move to the front and with your dominant hand open the student's hands flat while holding your non-dominant hand under the student's hands.

2. Draw Choku Rei in front of the student's third eye and silently chant Choku Rei three times as you picture it moving into the head though the third eye.

3. Draw Hon Sha Ze Sho Nen in front of the student's third eye and silently chant Hon Sha Ze Sho Nen three times as you picture it moving into the head though the third eye.

4. With your dominant hand draw Choku Rei in the air above the hands. Then picture the symbol moving into the hands as you silently chant Choku Rei three times. Pat the hands three times.

5. Bring the student's hands together and move them back to in front of the heart. Blow over the hands, up to the third eye and crown, back over the hands to solar plexus and back to the hands.

Complete the process with each student and continue to Part Three.

Part Three (back)
1. Place your hands on the student's shoulders and look down through the crown chakra imagining you can see into the heart chakra. Place a positive affirmation such as "You

are a successful and confident Reiki healer" or "Divine love and wisdom guides and empowers you in your use of Reiki" in the student's heart by silently repeating it three times, intending that it be accepted by the subconscious mind of the student.

2. Bring your hands together, placing your thumbs at the base of the skull. Repeat the phrase "I now seal this process with Divine love and wisdom" while picturing a door with Choku Rei on it being closed. While you do this intend, will and feel that the process is sealed and complete, and the student is now connected directly to the Reiki Source.

3. Place your palms on the student's shoulders and repeat the affirmation, "We are both blessed by this process" or hold this feeling for several seconds.

4. Move to the front. Ask the student(s) to place their hands palm down on their legs and to breathe deeply and slowly while opening her eyes. At this point you may add a final blessing of your own.

Fourth of Four Attunements

Part One (back)

1. Place both hands on top of the head and close your eyes, meditating briefly to gain energetic rapport with the student.

2. Draw the Usui Dai Ko Myo over the head while silently repeating "Dai Ko Myo" three times in mantra-like fashion. Picture the symbol moving into the crown chakra through the head and lodging in the base of the brain, guiding it with your dominant hand.

3. Draw Hon Sha Ze Sho Nen above the head while silently repeating "Hon Sha Ze Sho Nen" three times in mantra-like fashion. Picture the symbol moving into the crown chakra through the head and lodging in the base of the brain, guiding it with your dominant hand.

4. Draw Sei heki above the head while silently repeating Sei heki three times to yourself in mantra-like fashion. Picture the symbol moving into the crown chakra through the head and lodging in the base of the brain, guiding it with your dominant hand.

5. Reach over and move the student's prayer clasped hands to the top of her head.

6. Draw Choku Rei in the air above the hands. Picture the symbol moving into the hands and down into the crown chakra through the head and lodging in the base of the brain while silently chanting Choku Rei three times.

7. Gently move the student's hands from the top of their head directing them back down to in front of heart.

Complete the process with each student and continue to Part Two.

Part Two (front)

1. Move to the front and with your dominant hand, open the student's hands flat holding your non-dominant hand under the student's hands.

2. Draw Choku Rei in front of the student's third eye. Silently chant Choku Rei three times as you picture it moving into the head though the third eye.

3. Draw Hon Sha Ze Sho Nen in front of the student's third eye. Silently chant Hon Sha Ze Sho Nen three times as you picture it moving into the head though the third eye.

4. Draw Sei heki in front of the student's third eye. Silently chant Sei heki three times as you picture it moving into the head though the third eye.

5. With your dominant hand draw Choku Rei in the air above the hands. Picture the symbol moving into the hands as you silently chant Choku Rei three times. Pat the hands three times.

6. Bring the student's hands together and move them back in front of the student's heart. Blow over the hands, up to the third eye and crown, and back over the hands to the solar plexus and back to the hands.

Complete the process with each student and continue to Part Three.

Part Three (back)

1. Place your hands on the student's shoulders and look down through the crown chakra imagining that you can see into the heart chakra. Place a positive affirmation such as "You are a successful and confident Reiki healer" or "Divine love and wisdom guides and empowers you in your use of Reiki" in the student's heart by repeating it to yourself three times, intending that it be accepted by the subconscious mind by passing through the heart chakra of the student.

2. Bring your hands together, placing your thumbs at the base of the skull. Repeat the phrase "I now seal this process with Divine love and wisdom" while picturing a door with Choku Rei on it being closed and locked. While you do this intend, will and feel that the process is sealed and complete, and the student is now connected directly to the Reiki Source.

3. Place your palms on the student's shoulders and repeat the affirmation "We are both blessed by this process" or hold this feeling for several seconds.

4. Move to the front. Ask the student(s) to place their hands palm down on their legs and breathe deeply and slowly while opening their eyes. At this point you may add a final blessing of your own.

The Western/Takata System
Second Degree Attunement

You will be placing the Choku Rei, Sei heki and Hon Sha Ze Sho Nen into the hands for the Second Degree Attunement. This includes when they are on the head as well as when they are open in front. You will also be placing these symbols into the third eye. There is just one attunement for Reiki II.

Part One (back)

1. Place both hands on top of the head and close your eyes, meditating briefly to gain energetic rapport with the student.

2. Draw the Usui Dai Ko Myo over the head and while repeating Usui Dai Ko Myo three times to yourself in mantra-like fashion, picture the symbol moving into the crown chakra through the head and lodging in the base of the brain, guiding it with your right hand.

3. Reach over and move the student's prayer clasped hands to the top of his head.

4. Draw Choku Rei in the air over the hands. Then picture the symbol moving into the hands then down into the crown chakra through the head and lodging in the base of the brain while chanting Choku Rei to yourself three times.

5. Draw Sei heki in the air over the hands. Then picture the symbol moving into the hands then down into the crown chakra through the head and lodging in the base of the brain while chanting Sei heki to yourself three times.

6. Draw Hon Sha Ze Sho Nen in the air over the hands. Then picture the symbol moving into the hands then down into the crown chakra through the head and lodging in the base of the brain while chanting Hon Sha Ze Sho Nen to yourself three times.

7. Gently move the student's hands from the top of their head motioning them back down in front of heart.

Move on to the next person and repeat above, or if only one student, move to the front and do Part Two.

Second Degree Attunement

Part Two (front)

1. Move to the front and open the student's hands flat holding your non-dominant hand under the student's hands.

2. Draw Choku Rei in front of the student's third eye, then chant Choku Rei three times as you picture it moving into the head though the third eye.

3. Do step 2 with Sei heki and Hon Sha Ze Sho Nen so that you place all three symbols into the third eye.

4. With your dominant hand draw out Choku Rei in the air above the hands. Then picture the symbol moving into the hands as you chant to yourself Choku Rei three times. Then pat the hands three times.

5. Do step 4 with the Sei heki and Hon Sha Ze Sho Nen so that you place all three symbols into the hands.

6. Bring the student's hands together and move them back in front of the student's heart. Blow over the hands, up to the third eye, and crown, and back over the hands to solar plexus and back to hands.

Move to next the student and repeat above or go to Part Three.

Part Three (back)

1. Place your hands on the student's shoulders and look down through the crown chakra imagining you can see into the student's heart chakra. Place a positive affirmation in the student's heart by repeating it to yourself three times, intending it to be accepted by the subconscious mind by passing through the heart chakra of the student such as "You are a successful and confident Reiki healer" or "Divine love and wisdom guides and empowers you in your use of Reiki."

2. Bring your hands together, placing your thumbs at the base of the skull. Repeat the phrase "I now seal this process with Divine love and wisdom" while picturing a door with Choku Rei on it being closed and locked. While you do this, intend, will and feel that the process is sealed and complete and that the student is now connected directly to the Reiki source.

3. Place your palms on the student's shoulders and repeat the affirmation "We are both blessed by this process" or hold this feeling for several seconds.

4. Move to the front. Ask the student(s) to place their hands palm down on their legs and to breathe deeply and slowly while opening their eyes. You may add a final blessing of your own choosing if you are so inclined at this point.

The Western/Takata System
Third Degree Master Attunement

You will be placing all four Usui symbols into the hands and third eye for the Third Degree Attunement. This includes when they are on the head as well as when they are open in front.

Part One (back)

1. Place both hands on top of the head and close your eyes meditating briefly to gain energetic rapport with the student.

2. Reach over and move the student's prayer clasped hands to the top of her head.

3. Draw the Usui Dai Ko Myo over the hands and while repeating "Dai Ko Myo" three times to yourself in mantra-like fashion, picture the symbol moving through the hands into the crown chakra through the head and lodging in the base of the brain, guiding it with your dominant hand.

4. Do step 2 with the Choku Rei, Sei heki, and Hon Sha Ze Sho Nen.

5. Gently move the student's hands from the top of their head motioning them back down in front of heart.

Move on to the next person and repeat above or if only one student, move to the front and do Part Two.

Part Two (front)

1. Move to the front and open the student's hands flat holding your non-dominant hand under the student's hands.

2. Draw the Usui Master symbol in front of the student's third eye, then chant Dai Ko Myo, the Usui Master symbol, three times as you picture it moving into the head though the third eye.

3. Do step 2 with the Choku Rei, Sei heki, and Hon Sha Ze Sho Nen so that you place all four symbols into the third eye.

4. With your dominant hand draw out the Usui Dai Ko Myo in the air above the hands. Then picture the symbol moving into the hands as you chant to yourself Dai Ko Myo three times. Then pat the hands three times.

5. Do step 4 with the Choku Rei, Sei heki, and Hon Sha Ze Sho Nen so that you place all four symbols into the hands.

6. Bring the student's hands together and move them back in front of the student's

heart. Blow over the hands, up to the third eye, and crown, and back over the hands to solar plexus and back to hands.

Move to next the student and repeat above or go to Part Three.

Part Three (back)

1. Place your hands on the student's shoulders and look down through the crown chakra imagining you can see into the student's heart chakra. Place a positive affirmation in the student's heart by repeating it to yourself three times, intending it to be accepted by the subconscious mind by passing through the heart chakra of the student such as "You are a successful and confident Reiki healer" or "Divine love and wisdom guides and empowers you in your use of Reiki."

2. Bring your hands together, placing your thumbs at the base of the skull. Repeat the phrase "I now seal this process with Divine love and wisdom" while picturing a door with Choku Rei on it being closed. While you do this, intend, will and feel that the process is sealed and complete and that the student is now connected directly to the Reiki source.

3. Place your palms on the student's shoulders and repeat the affirmation "We are both blessed by this process" or hold this feeling for several seconds.

4. Move to the front. Ask the student(s) to place their hands palm down on their legs and to breathe deeply and slowly while opening their eyes. You may add a final blessing of your own choosing if you are so inclined at this point.

Alternate Western/Takata Reiki I Attunement

As stated previously, there are several methods in use for doing the Western style Usui/Takata attunements. The following is another method for doing the Usui Reiki I attunement. It is included in this manual so you will have additional information about another system currently in use. It is not intended for you to use this technique as a Center Licensed Reiki Teacher when teaching Reiki classes.

This is a First Degree Initiation done with four attunements and comes from the Furumoto lineage. Since this is a Western/Takata attunement it does not include the Tibetan symbols, the Violet Breath or contracting the Hui Yin.

1. Move behind the student and draw Choku Rei vertically above the head while silently repeating its name three times.

2. Draw Hon Sha Ze Sho Nen vertically starting at the top of the head and going down the back while silently repeating its name three times.

3. Draw Choku Rei horizontally above the top of the head and silently repeat its name three times.

4. Place your dominant hand on top of the student's head and the other hand upright in the air.

5. Silently repeat "Hon Sha Ze Sho Nen" three times and "Dai Ko Myo" three times in mantra-like fashion. (This is a mantra used many times throughout the attunement process.)

6. For Attunement One do seven sets of the mantra. For Attunements Two to Four do three sets of the mantra.

7. For the Fourth Attunement only, move the non-dominant hand to the base of the skull to seal. Repeat the mantra in step #5 three times. Wait for energy to equalize between the hands.

8. For the Second to Fourth Attunements place your hands on the student's shoulders and say the mantra three times.

9. Move to the front and draw Choku Rei with your dominant hand over the student's hands while they are in the prayer position. Say silently "Choku Rei" three times. Hold the student's hands with your hands so that the thumb of your dominant hand is folded over the top of the student's fingers and say the mantra three times. Then place the fingers of your dominant hand between the student's hands with the thumb of your dominant hand still folded over the top of the student's fingers and say the mantra three times.

10. Move the student's prayer-clasped hands up to the third eye so that the student's thumb is in line with the third eye.

11. Draw a large Choku Rei in front of the torso and silently say "Choku Rei" three times.

12. Draw Choku Rei with the tongue on the roof of the mouth, and silently say its name three times as you blow over the fingertips and top of the head.

13. Repeat step #12 with the heart chakra and solar plexus.

14. Move the student's hands down to their original position in front of the heart.

15. Draw Choku Rei over the forehead and silently say its name three times. Place your dominant hand horizontally, directing it to the third eye with the non-dominant hand going up into the air. Picture Choku Rei going into the head.

16. Remove your hand from the forehead and draw a large Choku Rei in front of the student to close. Bring your hands down to your sides to close the energy.

Usui/Tibetan
Four Attunement Method for Reiki I

In the Western/Takata Style attunement technique four attunements are given for First Degree Reiki. Experimentation has determined that because the Tibetan symbols and processes have been added to the Usui attunement technique, only one attunement as outlined in this manual is necessary to fully initiate a student into First Degree Reiki. If you wish to use four attunements for First Degree do the following:

In Attunement One do not use the Sei heki or Hon Sha Ze Sho Nen, but bring the hands up right after the Usui Dai Ko Myo is placed. Then place only Choku Rei in the hands while they are on top of the head.

In Attunement Two, Part One, place Sei heki into the crown after the Usui Dai Ko Myo and before the hands come up. Then place only Choku Rei into the hands while they are on the head.

In Attunement Three, place Hon Sha Ze Sho Nen into the crown after the Usui Dai Ko Myo and before the hands come up. Then place only Choku Rei into the hands while they are on the head.

In Attunement Four, place both Sei heki and Hon Sha Ze Sho Nen into the crown after the Usui Dai Ko Myo is placed and before the hands come up. Then place only Choku Rei into the hands while they are on the head. Remember, only Choku Rei is placed in the hands in all four attunements. Everything else is done exactly the same.

Notes

Notes

Notes

Teaching Reiki

Becoming a Reiki Master

In the end we must consider that a Reiki Master isn't one who has mastered Reiki, but one who has allowed herself to be mastered by Reiki.

Reiki is a sacred practice that requires reverence and our greatest respect if we are to experience the deeper aspects of its value. The benefits of Reiki can be all-encompassing, not only giving us the ability to heal ourselves and others, which by itself is deeply meaningful, but also bringing guidance for our lives. Its unlimited nature can create opportunities for continual growth and unfoldment of our boundless potential. The ever increasing joy, peace and abundance that await those who sincerely pursue the path of Reiki are not only a blessing to be enjoyed, but also contain the healing the planet so dearly needs. Those who have been initiated into Reiki often feel this greater potential and aspire to continue to the Advanced and Master levels.

The desire to grow is inherent in simply being alive. As we look around ourselves and observe other living things, we can clearly see that all living things share the impulse to grow. Because this is what living things do, one could even say that the purpose of life is to grow and develop. Therefore, the desire to grow in one's Reiki potential is a natural expression of one's core essence and of life itself. If you feel this desire in your heart, honor and respect it. Doing so will fulfill an innate need.

Reiki - A Joyful Path

The joys of becoming a Reiki Master are many, and you don't necessarily have to teach in order for the Master training to be useful. The additional healing energy, symbols, techniques and knowledge will add value to your healing abilities. Treating yourself and treating others in person and at a distance will all be noticeably improved. The fact that you can pass Reiki on to friends and family is also a definite plus. Many take the Master training with just this in mind. However, if you ever decide to formally teach, you will be able to do so. As you take Reiki Master training and increase your personal vibration, it adds to the vibration of the whole planet!

One of the greatest joys of Reiki Mastership is teaching Reiki to others. Imagine the thrill of witnessing the members of your Reiki class receiving Reiki energy during the attunement and then, as you guide them in its use, sharing in their joy and amazement as they experience its gentle power flowing through them for the first time. As your students use Reiki to help family, friends and clients, a wonderful sense of spiritual connection will develop among all of you. Feelings of compassion and love for everyone will be strengthened as you merge with the Reiki consciousness and know more deeply than ever before that we all come from God and that we are all one in God.

What Is a Reiki Master?

The definition of a teaching Reiki Master according to the Center is anyone who has received the Master attunement and master symbol and who understands how to give all the attunements. In order to be considered a Reiki Master, one must also have taught Reiki to at least one other person. Those who have taken Reiki Master training but not taught Reiki to anyone would not qualify as Reiki Masters so far as the Center is concerned and should call themselves Reiki Master practitioners instead until they do begin to teach.

Master Training is a Serious Step

Becoming a Reiki Master is a serious step that requires definite preparation. One must first take Reiki I & II and Advanced Reiki Training (ART). Practice in using Reiki is absolutely necessary. Experience with the energy and using the symbols is a must. It is also necessary to meditate on your life purpose and decide if Reiki Mastership is in harmony with it. Then, it is important to study with a competent and compatible Reiki Master who will encourage and help you after you complete the training.

How to Find the Right Teacher

Before taking Reiki Master training, you should ask your prospective teacher exactly what you will be able to do after you are trained. Will you receive the complete training and be able to initiate others into all the degrees including full Reiki Master? Or will something be left out, requiring you to take additional sublevels or degrees and pay additional fees? Because of changes some have made to the system of Reiki, this is a very important question to ask. If you choose to study with one of the Center's Licensed Teachers, you will receive the complete Reiki Master training.

Becoming a Reiki Master implies the ability to initiate others into Reiki. Therefore, it is important to find a teacher who will spend time in class helping you practice the attunement processes used in the initiations. Ask potential teachers how much time is spent in class practicing the attunements, as some teachers spend little or none. Also ask them how much support they are willing to give you to begin teaching your own classes. This is important. Some Reiki Masters will have little interest in helping you get started, as they are afraid you will take students away from them. If you are serious about becoming a successful teaching Reiki Master, find a teacher who will openly support you in achieving your goals.

After taking the Master training and before teaching your first class, additional practice doing the attunements is important. This can be done on friends who already have Reiki. Ask them if they would like to be "attunement models" and let them know that the additional attunements will be beneficial for them and will refine and strengthen their Reiki energies. Most will gladly agree. If you can't find someone to practice on, you can use a teddy bear or a pillow to represent a person.

It will also be necessary to practice the talks, lectures and meditations you will be leading in class. Make outlines of your talks and practice reading them into a recorder. Listen to your talks and take notes on ways you can improve them. Then continue to practice until you are confident. Don't be afraid to use your outline in class. When teaching, relax and let the Reiki energy do the work.

If you have a sincere desire to help others and have taken the time to prepare, you should have no trouble attracting students. It is your attitude that creates the results you receive, so assume success and you will create success.

Treat Students with Great Respect

As a teaching Reiki Master it is important to treat your students with the greatest respect. Know that all have the spark of God within them. Never use subtle threats or withhold information to make your students dependent on you. Openly encourage all students to be connected to their own power and freedom of choice. What you create for others comes back to you. As you truly empower others, so will you be empowered. Trust in the abundance of the Universe and you will receive abundance. You will also be blessed with peace and joy.

Set a Good Example

When teaching Reiki to others, it is important to set a good example by being an authentic representative of Reiki energy. People cannot be so easily fooled by surface spirituality now. They want and need a real teacher who comes from experience and is working on her or his own deep healing. This requires one to meditate on the nature of Reiki energy and surrender to it. It is a continual process of working with all aspects of one's being that are out of step with Reiki energy and allowing the energy to heal them. We must seek to develop and express the qualities of love, compassion, wisdom, justice, cooperation, humility, persistence, kindness, courage, strength and abundance, as Reiki energy is all of these and more. It may seem

paradoxical, but it is true that a real Reiki Master is one who is always becoming a Reiki Master. Like life itself, it is a process of continual growth.

As you do this, you will realize sooner or later that there is more to Reiki than using it to heal yourself and others of specific problems. Reiki has a deeper purpose. In the same way that Reiki is able to guide healing energy when you are giving a session, Reiki can guide your life.

Your Life Purpose

There is a perfect plan for your life that has always been present and waiting for you. This plan is exactly what is good and right and healthy for you. This plan is not necessarily based on what your parents want for you, or what your friends or the culture says you need to do to be accepted. It is based on what will really make you happy. This plan is inside of you and comes from your core essence. Reiki can activate and help you follow this plan, which is your true spiritual path.

By treating yourself and others and by meditating on the essence of Reiki, you will be guided more and more by Reiki in making important decisions. Sometimes you will find yourself doing things that don't seem to make sense or conform to what you think you should be doing, and sometimes you will be guided to do things that you have told yourself you would never do. However, by trusting more and more in the guidance of Reiki, by letting go of what your ego thinks it needs to be happy and by humbly surrendering to Reiki's loving power, you will find your life changing in ways that bring greater harmony and feelings of real happiness.

The Way of Reiki

Over time, you will learn from experience that the guidance of Reiki is worthy of your trust. Once you have surrendered completely, you will have entered The Way of Reiki. When you do this, you will be at peace with the past, have complete faith in the future and know that there never was anything to worry about. Your life will work with ever-greater harmony, and you will feel that you have reached your goal of wholeness even as you continue to move toward it!

In the end, we must consider that a Reiki Master is not one who has mastered Reiki, but one who has allowed Reiki to master him or her. This requires that we surrender completely to the spirit of Reiki, allowing it to guide every area of our lives and become our only focus and source of nurturing and sustenance.

As we proceed into the new millennium, The Way of Reiki offers itself as a solution to our problems and as a path of unlimited potential. May all who would benefit from this path be guided to it.

What Is Possible for a Reiki Master

Because of the nature of the Master level and the energies that become available to us, being a Reiki Master can be an ongoing process involving continuous personal growth. With the master attunement and the use of the master symbol, we receive the opportunity to open more and more completely to the limitless potential of Reiki and to develop in ourselves the qualities that are contained in the Reiki energy. Considering all the aspects of Reiki energy, besides the potential to heal virtually all illness, it also contains unlimited love, joy, peace, compassion, wisdom, abundance and even more. We know these are the qualities of Reiki because people experience them when giving or receiving Reiki sessions. They are especially apparent when we meditate on the source of Reiki.

When doing so, many are lifted up into a safe place where they feel completely cared for and where they become aware of the wonderful possibilities that can come from within. When we contemplate these things, it is easy to become filled with optimism and the confident understanding that all challenges in life can be met and that our lives can be a glorious experience.

The Japanese name for the Master level of Reiki is Shinpiden, which means "Mystery Teaching." The mystery that is spoken of here is the mystery of God's love, wisdom and power. It is a mystery because God has no boundaries; all the attributes of God including wonder, beauty and grace extend far beyond our ability to comprehend. No matter how developed we become in this life or in any future level of existence, we will never fully understand it. This is why it is and will always remain a wonderful mystery. When we receive the Usui Dai Ko Myo and the attunement that empowers it, we have created the possibility for us to become aware of the Ultimate Reality. This is expressed in the definition of the Usui Dai Ko Myo, which indicates that it represents that part of the self that is already completely enlightened! When we use the master symbol, we are actually connecting with our own enlightened selves. This, in fact, is the true source of Reiki energy—it actually comes from the deepest and most important part of our own nature—our own enlightened self, which is part of the God-Consciousness! While it may appear to some to come from outside us, appearing to come down through the crown chakra, this is actually an illusion and only appears this way because of our limited awareness.

Reiki comes to us by the Grace of God and it is this same Grace that heals us and fosters our personal growth. Yet development does not take place automatically. Reiki respects our free will and does not force development on us. But if we seek it and intend it, and use Reiki for this purpose, then certainly, we will be guided into a greater healing experience.

Experiment in Surrender

Try this experiment. Begin doing Reiki on yourself using the Usui Dai Ko Myo with your hands in any position that is comfortable. Then meditate on this affirmation. "I surrender completely to the Reiki energy and to God, which is

121

its source." Repeat this affirmation over and over, and then as the Reiki energy continues to flow, with your inner eye, look for the source of Reiki, either within yourself or above. By doing this, you will have many important experiences. These are likely to include becoming more aware of how Reiki is working within you, and feeling its amazing qualities. New possibilities for personal growth will be presented, and you will be invited to participate in life in a more meaningful way. As your awareness moves closer and closer to the source, you will become aware of amazing insights and have ever increasing experiences of joy, security and peace. This is a wonderful exercise and well worth the time. I suggest you do this every day and as you do so, these experiences will become stronger. Then, if you choose to accept the healing changes that are presented, deep healing will begin taking place, and you will also begin receiving guidance about how to improve your life. While this meditation is simple, it is also very powerful and can lead you into a very happy and healthy state of mind, creating lasting changes that will form the foundation of a more worthwhile life.

Reiki can guide you in ways to make its healing power more beneficial and to heal more deeply. And at the same time, it is possible that Reiki will guide you to other healing techniques that are exactly right for you to use in addition to Reiki. You may also receive guidance about changes you need to make that require you to take action. Your ability to make decisions will improve, making it very easy to decide exactly what you need, whom to associate with, where to work, and more. This meditation can result in an entirely new direction for your life!

When you are involved in the healing process, a good way to determine your progress is to use your outer world as an indication of your inner development. This works because we manifest our entire experience through our thoughts and intentions both conscious and unconscious. When we experience something in our lives, it is because some part of our being has created it. When we accept this idea and take complete responsibility for what takes place in our lives, we enter a very powerful place. We can then change the things that are not healthy and improve every aspect of our lives. If your outer world contains positive experiences, and you are enjoying your life, this means that your inner world is in a similar state. The reverse is also true. When we experience painful things or are disappointed or experience things that foster fear, worry or doubt, this is also because some part of our inner being is out of balance and needs healing. If something unpleasant or unwanted takes place in your life, rather than blaming other people or circumstances outside yourself, direct your attention inward and look for the part of yourself that has created this unpleasant event. Then use your Reiki healing skills to nurture and heal this part. When you do this, the unpleasant experiences will stop and be replaced by healthy positive experiences. (Use of the *Healing Your Shadow Self* CD can be helpful with this process.)

As we continue on our healing path, we become aware of a level of consciousness that resides deeply within each of us that brings a wonderful new way of living. It creates a new attitude that is entirely positive and carries with it the ability to solve many problems and create positive results that previously we did not think possible. This higher consciousness is what the saints, holy people and those upon whom religions have been founded experienced, and it is what allowed them to perform miracles. This new consciousness is coming to many people now and in a short time will become the normal state for most of the people on earth. This is actually a higher aspect of Reiki consciousness. It is becoming more and more available to all of us. In fact, this higher way of manifesting our lives has been part of the highest aspects of all religious practice and has gone by many names, depending on which religious or spiritual group named it. A breakthrough like this is possible with Reiki, so I encourage you to accept this possibility and work with it.

Let us release all desire to hold onto negative ways that limit our happiness, and instead, embrace the inner light of Reiki. Within the source of Reiki resides the love of the universe. Those who focus on this love, and surrender to its healing power are opening to wonderful changes that will lead not only to peace within, but also to peace on earth.

A worthy goal for all Reiki Masters is to become the kind of Reiki Master you yourself would have liked to have had as a teacher when you were taking Reiki classes.

The Promise of a Thriving Reiki Practice

People come to you with many different problems, difficulties and illnesses, sometimes as a last resort, and you watch them leave relaxed, often radiant with joy and new hope...seeing them improve over time, watching them grow, gain confidence and become more trusting of life...seeing some make major changes and life adjustments...occasionally witnessing miracles...feeling the wonder of God's love pass through you and into another...sensing the presence of spiritual beings, feeling their touch, and knowing they work with you...being raised into ever greater levels of joy and peace by simply placing your hands on another...watching your life grow and develop as your continual immersion in Reiki transforms your attitudes, values and beliefs...sensing that because of your commitment to help others, beings of light are focusing their love and healing on you and carefully guiding you on your spiritual path. All this is the promise of a thriving Reiki practice!

Create a Thriving Reiki Practice, Part I
Vision, Intention and Attitudes

By William Lee Rand

If you've taken a Reiki class, even if it is Level I, it's possible to use your skill as a healer to start a Reiki practice. That's right; you don't need to wait until you've become a Reiki Master to start a practice. Back in the 80's, when Reiki II cost $500 and only a select few could become Reiki Masters, it was considered normal and appropriate to start an active Reiki practice after taking the first class. Keep in mind that Takata Sensei worked in Dr. Hayashi's clinic giving professional Reiki sessions to his clients with only Reiki I training.

Remember, you're not the one doing the healing; it's the Reiki energy. Its supply is unlimited, and it is guided by the highest Divine wisdom. How could you doubt

taken one of the higher degrees, that is even better, but the important thing is that if you have any level of training, as long as it was good training, you're ready to start right now.

There is tremendous value in having a thriving Reiki practice. Think about what this would look and feel like. If you had 10 clients a week and charged $75 each, you'd be earning close to $40,000 a year just from sessions. You'd likely be working 10-15 hours a week giving the sessions and an additional 10 or so hours for marketing, bookkeeping and other business activities for a total of about 25 hours a week! You'd even be able to work from your home if you wanted to. How

In the development of a thriving Reiki practice, issues, problems and challenges are bound to arise. When this happens, always remember to call on Reiki to guide you through them. There will likely be something within yourself needing to heal.

that it wouldn't work right or provide the healing your clients need? One of the most important lessons the beginning Reiki practitioner or practitioners at any level can learn is to have confidence in the Reiki energy to guide you in creating the healing experience that is exactly right for each client. When you are able to set your ego aside and trust that Reiki will work, you are ready to become a Reiki practitioner. And this can be done even after taking a beginning class! In saying this, I'm talking about someone who has taken a well-organized class from a competent instructor and has also taken the time to practice by giving complete sessions with friends and family. If you've

do those numbers sound? If you decided to teach, which wouldn't be difficult with that kind of clientele as potential students, you could add an additional $20,000 or more to your income. As you can see, a Reiki practice can be a real job that earns real income. There is also a special satisfaction that comes from being your own boss and running your own business.

In addition to these purely financial results, there are also emotional and spiritual benefits that can be even more fulfilling. You'll be immersed in Reiki energy several hours a day on a regular basis. This will have a positive affect on your health. At the same time, giving Reiki sessions to others and seeing them heal and grow will fill your heart with peace and joy. You'll be providing a service to others and to your community that will connect you to them in a very loving and spiritual way. Being in this type of energetic environment will quicken your personal growth and move you more quickly along on your spiritual path.

As you can see, a successful Reiki practice can provide you with both material and spiritual benefits in a way that is entirely healthy for you and your clients. Getting a successful practice started will require a clear commitment and focused activity over a period of time. Starting out with a part time effort and eventually working at it full time, it might take six months or more of promoting and developing your practice before you begin to approach the numbers mentioned above, but a thriving Reiki practice provides rewards that are more than worth the effort it takes to create success. Think about how valuable a successful practice will be for you, your life and for those who come to see you for sessions.

The first step toward realizing your goal is to do an assessment of your inner attitudes and beliefs as well as the personal resources you possess that can be employed in the attainment of your goal.

The foundation of all we do is our inner state. It is out of this state that we are able to create what we attempt to do. Having a strong enthusiastic intention to achieve your goal is necessary. If you have a half-hearted desire or are not really excited about creating a thriving Reiki practice, or if you don't really believe you can do it,

or if you feel that you don't really deserve it, then you're not likely to do very well. It takes strong motivation backed by emotional energy to achieve a goal as important as this. If you don't have this state spontaneously, or if you find yourself in a slump once you've started your project, there is something you can do to pump yourself back up. Here's an exercise that is important to do right from the beginning and continue everyday. It will give you the energy and enthusiasm you need to accomplish your goal.

Goal Manifesting Exercise

1. Write your goal on a 3x5 card something like this: "I have a thriving Reiki practice. I see ten or more clients a week and teach classes. I have a thriving Reiki practice. I see ten or more clients a week and teach classes. I have a thriving Reiki practice. I see ten or more clients a week and teach classes." Be sure to repeat it three times.

2. Then place the card in your hand. If you've taken Reiki II or higher, draw all your Reiki symbols in the air over the card. If not, then simply use Reiki by itself.

3. Place the card between your hands and give it Reiki, intending that the Reiki energy empower and manifest your goal.

4. As you do this, repeat the affirmation to yourself over and over as you send it Reiki.

5. In addition, visualize yourself with a thriving Reiki practice. Picture this imagery in a field of Reiki light up above your head. See yourself looking at your client file and seeing it full of client records. See checks and money flowing into your pocket

and your bank account. See yourself in your treatment room working with a client knowing many more are on the way. When you visualize this, know in your heart that when this happens, it will be a truly exciting and satisfying accomplishment. Fill yourself with feelings of excitement, joy and success as though it's actually happening right now! Allow yourself to get caught up in this inner state so that you lose awareness of your surroundings and are as fully absorbed as possible in the positive feelings of having a thriving Reiki practice.

6. Do this exercise at least once a day, but more often if possible. The more you do it, the better you'll be able to enter the desired state and the more beneficial it will be for you.

This exercise is very important to practice everyday. It is part of the training you need to strengthen your energy field and cultivate the inner qualities necessary to excel at accomplishing your purpose. It is better if you do it at the same time each day, such as in the morning before you start your day or at lunchtime. Not only will it give you the personal energy to accomplish your goal and motivate you to do what you need to do, it will enhance your creativity and create a powerful magnetic force that will attract to you all the people and resources you need. This will make it much easier to develop a thriving Reiki practice.

Because Reiki energy is the basis of this process, you'll be developing a special connection to the highest level of guidance and healing. This connection will develop over time to be a wonderful source of strength, inspiration and encouragement that will help you develop all the personal qualities necessary to accomplish and even surpass your goals.

Business Consciousness

Since Reiki is a spiritual practice, some of you may have a feeling, either consciously acknowledged or lurking around in the subconscious, that spiritual things and the material world don't belong together. If this feeling is present, it needs to be dealt with and healed. There is nothing wrong with the spiritual and material working together. In fact, that's the whole purpose for spiritual beings (you and me) to be in material bodies—to bring the values and energy of the spiritual world into the material world. Having a spiritual business is an excellent way to accomplish this purpose.

Often a person may be a great healer but does not do well because they haven't taken the time to develop the necessary business skills. In fact some practitioners actually shun the business aspect and then complain that they aren't making any money. This doesn't make sense. Remember, if you charge money for what you do and what you do is helping others, the better your business operates, the more people you'll be able to help, and this will directly affect your income. So don't shy away from the fact that you charge money and that you are a business person. You need to fully embrace it and be the best business person you can be.

Remember, regardless of your current knowledge or skill level, you can always improve. So even if you don't think you have the aptitude, it's important to take the time to learn and get the business aspect of your operation set up as well as you can. Some basic things you'll need are a set of books to record income and expenses and a marketing program. I'll discuss more about this in Part II of this article.

In setting up and operating your Reiki business, it's important to keep the spiritual and material in balance and working together in harmony. In your business practices, always make sure you are honest and fair in all you do and that your primary motivation is to sincerely help your clients. As your income goes up, you'll be able to expand your program and provide more services, thus helping even more people.

Money Issues

Since you're charging money for Reiki sessions and classes, your relationship to money will have a lot to do with how successful you become. Our culture seems to have a love-hate relationship with money. Remember, money is not good or bad in itself. It's no different than any other tool you might have. Think of a match. A match can be used to light a fire to cook your food or to burn down a house. Money is the same way. It's not what money is that counts, but what you do with it. If you earn your money honestly by providing services that people value and if you save and spend it wisely, then you'll be using money in a healthy way that is in alignment with the energy and principles of Reiki.

Since money is a major issue for most people, it's important for you to look at how you feel about money and heal any issues that come up. Here are some thought experiments. Try them out. You may not get negative feelings

from these exercises, but if you do, it's important to think about and heal them by including the issues in your regular self-healing sessions.

Money Thought Experiment

1. How do you feel when you find out someone else might be making more money than you?
2. How do you feel when you realize that you're making more money than someone else?
3. Think about how much money you're making right now. Then think what it would be like to make twice as much or three times as much. Do you feel like you are balancing on the top of a pole, afraid you're going to fall off? Are you afraid some one is going to take your money from you or that it will be difficult to hang onto?

If you want to have a successful Reiki business, it's important for you to be connected to money in a healthy way that empowers you to establish your spiritual values in the material world. If the above thought exercises bring up unhealthy feelings, or if other experiences with money cause unhealthy feelings, it's important that you acknowledge them and heal them. Doing this will create the necessary foundation for you to live a healthy and prosperous life.

Competition

An issue that is likely to come up in your Reiki practice is competition from other Reiki practitioners. Your understanding and your attitude toward competition will play an important role in how you deal with it and how it affects your Reiki practice. Fear of competition has caused more problems and restrictions for Reiki practitioners than any other issue. This fear is based on the illusion that there isn't enough for everyone, that another Reiki teacher will take your clients or students or that if there are too many Reiki practitioners in your area, then you'll have fewer clients. Remember, FEAR is really False Evidence Appearing Real. This is especially true for Reiki. It is the fear of competition that causes problems, not competition itself.

It's important to always maintain a healthy, positive attitude toward other Reiki practitioners and teachers. If you fear them or are jealous of them or have other negative feelings toward them, then your vibration will be lowered and this will cause you to attract fewer clients. Fear of competition tends to be self-fulfilling.

There is an important lesson about this topic we can learn from Reiki. Reiki energy comes from an unlimited supply. Because of this, we'll never run out of Reiki energy, no matter how many people are giving Reiki sessions. The reason Reiki is unlimited is that it comes from a higher level of consciousness. As long as we come from a higher level of consciousness when we plan and carry out our business activities, we'll be able to tap into this same unlimited supply which will result in abundance and prosperity in our lives.

Remember, potential Reiki clients and students are sensitive to energy. They also know that Reiki is a spiritual practice. They are looking for a practitioner/teacher who has a high vibration and who lives by spiritual values. If you have negative feelings toward other Reiki practitioners, potential customers will easily detect

your attitude, and they'll tend not to be attracted to you. This will also happen subconsciously, as those interested in Reiki usually have a higher intuitive sense and will be guided away from those with a lower vibration. Therefore, it's important for you to deal with any negative feelings that come up within you and heal them. Always say positive things about other Reiki people or say nothing at all.

Reiki is guided by the highest spiritual wisdom, and it also works in other ways by guiding clients and students to the right teacher. Those who are on spiritual paths or who are seeking healing often receive help from spirit guides who are on the lookout for the right Reiki practitioners for them. Therefore it's important to maintain a high spiritual vibration and to have the attitude that no one can take students or clients away from you, and you're not taking them from other Reiki practitioners, but that all students and clients are guided to the teacher or practitioner that is right for them. This will keep you in alignment with the Reiki energy and with the highest spiritual forces that are guiding the healing community.

It's also important that the primary motivation for your Reiki practice be to truly help your clients and students. If you are overly focused on money or have a need to control others, prospective clients/students will notice this, and they will not be attracted to you. Their spirit guides will recognize this attitude even more readily and will be less likely to guide them to you. Because of this, it's really important to be clear about your motivation. A good question to ask yourself is why you want to have a thriving Reiki business. While there may be a number of good reasons, the primary one that will really work is that you truly want to help people.

Some Reiki teachers have attempted to get their students to sign non-competitive agreements indicating that they won't teach in their territory. Others have declared that a certain area is their territory and that other teachers can't practice there. Again, this tactic is based on fear and ends up having the opposite affect than what was intended. The teacher usually ends up with less business because the energy of fear and control repels potential students and clients. Also, it's important to think in terms of how Reiki might think of a situation like this. If Reiki is focused on providing benefit to the client or student, wouldn't it be better if clients and students had more choices for potential teachers and practitioners? If you're in a situation where you're being told that you're in someone else's territory, send Reiki to the situation and follow the guidance you receive. Make sure that you respond in a way that maintains your high vibrational state and honors the values of Reiki. Remember, unless some prior agreement has been made, there are no territories in the Reiki world.

It's been found that when Reiki teachers and practitioners work together to promote Reiki, rather then competing with each other, they create a vortex of positive energy that is a much stronger attractive force than each of them working separately. This was demonstrated by Laurelle Shanti Gaia and Kathie Lipinski while they were practicing Reiki in Louisville, Kentucky. (See "Creating Harmony in the Reiki Community" in the Reiki Articles section at www.reiki. org) They organized teachers in their area who were competing with each other in negative ways and got them to work together in harmony. This may seem like a daunting task, but they called on Reiki to help and had the courage to follow their guidance. It worked! Because their group, called *United In Healing*, had so many members, they were able to organize events they wouldn't have been able to create on their own. They networked with support groups for breast cancer, fibromyalgia, diabetes and other chronic illnesses. They sponsored Reiki marathons for critically and chronically ill people and had a free clinic. In one weekend, their members had over 102 students in Reiki classes. This was a real blessing to the teachers and especially to the students and the community.

If you maintain a positive mental attitude toward members of the Reiki community in your area, your connection to Reiki will remain strong, which will allow the wisdom of Reiki to continue guiding you. This will make it easy to meditate with Reiki requesting insight on how to manage your business and how to improve it so as to attract more business, so that rather than competing, you can focus on creating. Remember, the purpose of Reiki and of your Reiki business is to provide benefit to your clients and students. If you're not getting the results you'd like, then place your focus on creating greater benefits for your clients and students. Develop your Reiki practice by taking more training to enhance your healing abilities, improving your teaching skills and the way your classes are organized, revising and upgrading your class manuals, promotional brochures, and web site, or develop new teaching aids and marketing ideas. This is the positive way to deal with competition; improve your business.

In the development of a thriving Reiki practice, issues, problems and challenges are bound to arise. When this happens, always remember to call on Reiki to guide you through them. There will likely be something within yourself needing to heal. As you heal and release your inner issues, the outer issues will be resolved as well. This is the miracle of Reiki. As you focus on helping others you also benefit. And as this process unfolds, your Reiki business can turn into an important part of your spiritual path.

Part II will focus on practical ways to develop and market your Reiki practice. Before reading part II of this article I suggest you read this article again and practice the Goal Manifesting Exercise and the Money Thought Experiment along with really using the ideas in this article and giving yourself Reiki for any issues that come up. By doing so you'll have strengthened your foundation and be ready for the practical application that I'll be sharing with you in part II.

Create a Thriving Reiki Practice, Part II

By William Lee Rand

Part I of this article (Winter 2006) focused on developing your state of mind. This is the most important part of creating a thriving Reiki practice because everything you create originates in your mind. The quality of the thoughts and feelings that surround your goals determines your likelihood of achieving them. The clearer you create your images of success and the stronger you believe in them, the more directly you'll be manifesting your goals with your mind. To say it another way: the mind is like a broadcasting station, sending out a signal that tells the Universe what to create for you. If you believe that creating a Reiki practice will be hard and that you're not likely to get many clients, this is what the Universe will create for you. On the

techniques and methods presented here have been tested and proven to work. But you must understand that each person and each situation is different and may require a unique combination of these methods or the development of methods not mentioned here.

Here is a formula for success. If followed carefully, it will guide you to the achievement of your goals.

1. Clearly decide on your goal. This must be stated in a concrete way using numbers and dates. As an example, you might decide your goal is to average 10 Reiki clients per week within four months.

The Secret of Success

I began saying a prayer right after I received my Reiki I training. I said this prayer sincerely everyday. It guided me to be a Reiki master and inspired me to develop my Reiki practice. It has continually created miraculous results in my life. The prayer is: **Guide me and heal me so that I might be of greater service to others.**

other hand, if you believe that creating a thriving Reiki practice will be easy and that you're going to have an abundant number of clients, then this is what the Universe will create for you. This is the inner marketing aspect of your business, and *it must come first*. Only by believing in yourself and the worthiness of your goals will you be able to convince others to do the same. So, if you haven't read Part I, I suggest you read it and put into practice the exercises it contains.

Assuming you are developing your inner marketing program, you can now start your outer marketing program. The ideas,

2. Develop a plan and follow it. Remember – those that fail to plan, plan to fail. Base your plan on methods others have used to achieve similar goals. The methods mentioned in this article are a good place to start. Remember to meditate with Reiki energy when contemplating the use of a particular method and in developing your plans. Reiki will guide you in miraculous ways and open doors you didn't know were there.

3. As you implement your plan, keep a record of the results you get. Note what methods work best to move

you toward your goal. Also note which ones don't work or produce poor results. It is important not to guess; keep records and look at the numbers.

4. Keep doing the things that work. Stop doing the things that don't work.

5. By eliminating the things that don't work, you'll have additional time and resources. Use them to try new things.

This may appear to be a very simple formula—because it is. Achieving success isn't a complicated process. It's just a matter of doing the right things consistently until you reach your goal. Note that even though it's a simple formula, each step is important and must be followed. As you follow this plan, over time you will develop a powerful set of business practices that move you toward your goal quickly and efficiently.

Reiki Room

You'll need a place to give your Reiki sessions. You can use a room in your home or rent an office. An office gives a more professional appearance and is a demonstration of your commitment. It is an additional business expense, but it can be cost effective by attracting more clients. However, if you can't afford it at the beginning or if you're guided to do so, it's also possible to set up a room in your home to give sessions.

You will need a Reiki table, a CD player, a couple of chairs, a table and a small filing cabinet for your records. Soft lighting, candles and incense are often helpful to create ambiance. The more relaxing and comfortable your Reiki room is, the more receptive your clients will be to the healing work you do.

Liability Insurance

I've never heard of anyone being sued for a bad Reiki session, but liability insurance can still be a good idea in some situations. Professional liability insurance will protect you if for some reason the client claims he or she was harmed by the Reiki session. The insurance company will legally represent you and negotiate with the client or defend you in court if necessary (even though this is unlikely to happen). However, the main reason to have it is that it is required by hospitals and medical clients if you should get the opportunity to give Reiki sessions there. While you usually won't receive pay for volunteering in a hospital or medical clinic, you will gain quality experience that will strengthen your professional credibility, enhance your bio, and likely increase the number of clients you have in your regular Reiki practice. It is also tremendously rewarding on an emotional and spiritual level.

General liability insurance is different from Professional liability insurance and is important for you to have. It will protect you if your client should fall off your Reiki table or if he or she slips and falls in your home or on the driveway in front of your home or in some other way becomes injured while on your property.

The Reiki Membership Association offers an excellent Reiki insurance program that includes both Professional and General liability for multiple modalities at an excellent price. Find out more at: http://www.reikimembership.com/Insurance.aspx or see page 144.

133

Records

There are various records you'll need to keep. These include:

1. Client records: I suggest using the Client Information Form that you can download free from our Web site: http://www.reiki.org/Download/FreeDownloads.html. This form informs the client that Reiki does not take the place of medical treatment. It is also a way to keep track of client contact information, as well as keeping a session history so you can check progress and see what techniques you have used and their results. It is also a way to collect email addresses for your email list, which is an important way to market your business.

2. Bookkeeping records: This can start out simply with a record book to keep track of expenses and income. You will also need a file for keeping expense receipts. You will need these for tax purposes, but it is also important to keep records to track the performance of your business and check your progress toward your goal.

Business Expenses are Tax Deductible

Because you are operating a business, you will be able to deduct business expenses from your income taxes, for which you will need records. Office rent, training expenses, including travel and lodging, as well as electricity, heat, gas for your car, and so forth may all be deducted from your taxes.

As your business expands, you may find it easier to use a computer accounting program. There are several that are free,

such as Microsoft Accounting Express 2007, and others, such as Intuit or QuickBooks, that charge a fee. Besides making your bookkeeping easier, they usually include other helpful features such as a contact manager that will allow you to create a list of all your clients and contact people and which usually includes an email list manager.

Marketing Tools

You need to promote your business by letting people know who you are and the services you offer. There are many ways to do this, and it is important to try as many as possible and track the results you get from each, so you can keep doing what works and stop doing what doesn't.

It is possible to start your Reiki business on a shoestring, and this may be the best way for many to get started, but at some point, it will be necessary to increase the amount of money you spend on marketing and promotion. This can be done gradually. As you get more clients, your income will grow, and it will be possible to expand your marketing program proportionally. When spending more on promotion, it's important to carefully track your results so you can keep doing the things that are cost effective and stop doing those that aren't. At the same time, it's important to keep in mind that there are many ways to promote your business that don't involve a lot of expense.

Email List

One of the most effective things you can do to promote your Reiki practice is develop an email list of those interested in Reiki. In today's world people use email to communicate far more than snail mail. This is because email is easy, fast and inexpensive. If you're promoting your Reiki practice, it's easier to compose an email and send it to your email list than to mail a flyer. With email, it's as easy as clicking a mouse button a few times, and it's done with almost no expense. With snail mail, it will take hours or days to get the mailing ready, and the expense can be in the hundreds or even thousands of dollars. Email is the way to go and results are almost instantaneous.

Because of this, it's important to begin collecting email addresses of those interested in Reiki right away. Collect them from your clients by having them fill in their email addresses on your Client Information Form and collect them from all the promotions and events you're involved with.

You can use your email list to remind people about your Reiki practice, let them know about promotions or special deals you have, or about your Free Reiki Evenings or Fund Raisers and so forth. *An effective email list is the most important marketing tool you can develop.*

Many email software programs allow you to send to a large list without the whole email list going to each recipient. There are bulk email Web sites that provide online software for sending out to large lists, and you can also get your own software programs and install them on your computer or on your Web server. Do a Google search for Bulk Email Service to locate providers. One email program I recommend is Subscribe Me Pro http://www.siteinteractive.com/subpro/ This program is only $49.00 and provides tracking.

To learn more about the importance of email for marketing I suggest you go to the Guerrilla Marketing Web site at www.gmarketing.com and read their article on email and marketing. You will also find other interesting articles there. I recommend you order the book, Mastering Guerrilla Marketing, which explains how to achieve your marketing goals with minimum expense.

Web Site

While a Web site isn't a necessity and you can start your Reiki practice without one, it's important to get a Web site as soon as possible to take advantage of its important marketing features. A Web site is a handy way to let people know what you do. Rather than trying to give a detailed verbal description of your services to people, or give them a bunch of handouts, just give them your Web address. They will have access to all of your material and be able to read through it at their leisure and return again and again until they convince themselves to come to you for a session. Also, the Web is such an integral part of society now that if you don't have a Web site, most people will think you're not serious about your business.

A well-designed Reiki Web site needs to contain:

1. An explanation of Reiki, including a Frequently Asked Questions section.
2. A description of your sessions, how long they last, your fee, etc. Testimonials from your clients are also a big plus.
3. If you're teaching, include a class schedule and a complete description of what each class contains, and what students will be able to do after taking each class. Class fees and prerequisites should also be listed.

4. A bio of yourself including a picture and especially your training background and experience.
5. Articles you have written about Reiki.
6. An email collection box to collect email addresses of visitors to your site.
7. Contact information including phone, email address, city and state, but not your home or business street address. Your exact location, including a map, can be sent separately to those who have scheduled a session or signed up for a class. This will prevent people from coming by without an appointment.

You can start out with a simple site that you design, but after a while, it's a good idea to have a professional Web master design and set up your Web site. Remember that people will determine who you are by the quality of the promotional material you provide. So make sure your Web site looks professional, is well organized, clearly communicates your ideas and provides useful information. One way to find a good Web master is to find Web sites online that you like and contact the Web masters of those sites to find out how much they charge for Web design, and get a feel for whether you can work with them, etc.

As I mentioned above, an important feature for your Web site is an email collection box. This provides a method for you to collect the email addresses of those who frequent your Web site. Subscribe Me Pro provides a method of setting this up. To get people to give you their email address, you'll need to offer them something. You could offer to give them a pod cast or recording of a Reiki talk or meditation you've recorded or to receive a free Reiki newsletter or

something of that nature. Be sure to place a value on what they'll get such as $5 or $10.

Business Cards

It's important to have a business card listing your name, phone and, especially, your email address and Web site, along with your business name, if you have one, and the Reiki services you offer. It's better not to list your street address to prevent people from coming to your office without an appointment. A business card lets people know you're serious and professional and makes it easy for people to contact you. Carry them with you at all times. You will be surprised at the number of opportunities to pass out your cards, especially when you're focused on the promotion of your Reiki practice.

Short Explanation of Reiki

Create short, succinct answers for basic Reiki questions so you'll be ready to explain Reiki to those who express interest. When people ask what Reiki is, I usually say; *"Reiki is a Japanese technique for relaxation that also promotes healing. It's done through touch. A warm and soothing energy flows from the hands into the client, promoting relaxation and releasing tension."* This answer usually inspires comments such as: "I could really use something like that." Or "Boy do we really need that around here." If you get a positive response like this, offer to give a short demo of five minutes or so to treat the person's shoulders or anywhere they may have tension or an ache or pain. Then give them a business card and answer any other questions they may have. They may contact you for a session or may refer others.

Impromptu Reiki Sessions

When you're out and about, talk to people, and weave the fact that you do Reiki into your conversation. If they ask what Reiki is, give them the short explanation above and offer to give them a short demo. Just place your hands on their shoulders to show them how the energy feels. Often they'll say things like, "I really need this," or "Wow that's going right for my sore arm," or "My headache is going away." Or you may be talking to someone and they mention an ache or pain they have. Immediately offer to give them Reiki for it. Many times, they'll already know what Reiki is, or if not, then give them your short explanation. Then let them know you do professional Reiki sessions and give them your card. You could also go on to explain how Reiki can help those undergoing chemotherapy and how it promotes healing after surgery and so forth. A hands-on experience like this will leave an impression, and even if they don't sign up for a session, they may refer others to you. Most will know of someone going into the hospital or in need of healing for one condition or another.

This technique is great at parties. You can either weave into your conversations that you do Reiki or those you talk with may offer that they have an ache or pain or a tense situation at work, which is a great lead-in for offering them Reiki. Once you start giving a demo session, often a crowd will gather, and you can give a little talk about Reiki to those watching as you give the treatment. Afterwards, pass out your business cards to those interested.

Upward Price Technique

If you are just starting a Reiki practice, try this technique for motivating people to come to you for sessions. When someone asks how much you charge, say, "I'm giving 10 sessions for free, and I've already given four (or whatever the number is at that point). Then say, "After the 10 free sessions, I'm going to be charging $10.00 per session." This will motivate people to sign up right away so they get a free session and avoid having to pay $10.00. After you've given out your 10 free sessions when someone asks how much you charge, say, "I'm giving 10 sessions for $10 each, and I've already given three (or whatever the number is at that point). After the 10, my price is going up to $20 per session." This will continue to motivate people to get sessions from you while the price is low. Continue with this process until you reach your target fee. By working like this, you'll be charging a fee based on your experience, and you will be motivating people to come to you quickly for sessions so they will save money.

Target Fee

Your target fee is the fee you want to work up to for Reiki sessions after you've gained experience, developed your business, and have a steady stream of clients. Your target fee will vary depending on the part of the country you live in. Doing a little research will help you figure this out. One way is to check with other experienced Reiki practitioners in your area to see what they charge. Another way is to set your target fee in the same range as professional massage therapists are charging in your area. Also remember that additional factors to consider when determining your target fee are the amount of training you've had, the amount of experience, and the results clients get from your sessions.

Clients Are Your Best Promoters

Those who have experienced your work are the best people to promote you. Make sure you give every client some of your business cards to hand out to friends, family and acquaintances who could use Reiki sessions.

Bonus Program

Creating a bonus program based on clients getting free sessions for bringing you new paying clients is also a way to promote your practice. When you give your clients business cards to pass out, tell them that for every two paying clients they send to you, you'll give them a free session. When clients come to you, you'll need to ask them how they found out about your practice and if anyone referred them to you. Use an Excel spreadsheet to keep track of how many each client referred to you. When a client gets the required number, email them and let them know they've earned a free session. Concerning the number they need to get a free session, remember that the idea is to build up your Reiki practice quickly and that each new client could become a promoter of your business too. Keeping the required number low will motivate them to work harder promoting your business.

Professional Referrals

Make friends with the chiropractors, massage therapists, acupuncturists, aroma therapists, medical doctors and other professionals in your area and let them know that you'll refer clients to them, if they'll refer clients to you. Collect business cards from them and give each some of yours. If they are hesitant to do this, offer them a free session, and then give them some of your cards to give to their clients. This method can also open the possibility of being offered a job giving sessions at a clinic.

Flyers

It's good to have a basic flyer to promote your business. Carry them with you to place on bulletin boards in health food stores, bookstores, churches, and so forth, and to give to prospective clients. Include a brief explanation of Reiki and the benefits it provides. If possible, include testimonials from your clients. Also be sure to create special flyers to reflect new promotions or services you're offering.

Magazine Advertising

I would be leaving out an important marketing method if I failed to mention advertising in the *Reiki News Magazine*. The magazine goes directly to 20,000 people who have a serious interest in Reiki, and it's a fact that those who advertise in our magazine get results. This is especially true for those who provide professional advertising copy and graphics and advertise regularly. If you want to find the ads that are working, check the current issue and then work your way through previous issues to see who's advertising consistently. The ads that appear in multiple issues are the ones that are working because people don't continue advertising unless it is cost effective.

Free Reiki Evening

This is also called a Reiki Share group and is an evening usually offered on a regular basis, such as once or twice a month, when Reiki practitioners get together to exchange Reiki. People who have never experienced Reiki can also be invited. Those who have Reiki training are asked to bring their Reiki tables. Usually a talk is given at the beginning that explains Reiki and answers questions. Usually, those new to Reiki receive sessions first, often with several practitioners giving them Reiki at the same time. A table can be set up for practitioners to display their business cards and flyers. Announcements about classes or other Reiki activities can also be made. Include a registration sheet to get names and email addresses to add to your email list so you can keep them notified about future Reiki events.

This is an excellent way to meet new Reiki practitioners, attract those seeking healing, and to advertise your practice. A subtle benefit of these meetings is that it keeps Reiki awareness high in your community and creates good will that will come back to you to support your practice. See *Reikishares* by Amy Rowland and Laurelle Gaia in the Spring 2005 issue of *Reiki News Magazine* for a complete description on how to set up and run a Reiki Share group.

Fundraisers

Non-profit organizations such as churches and charity groups often sponsor fundraising events. You could volunteer to set up and operate a Reiki fundraising event to benefit a group you wish to support. In this event, you provide free Reiki sessions and the clients give either a donation or a fixed fee to the organization. Be sure to create a sign-up sheet that includes the recipient's email address so you can add them to your email list. Explain on the sign-up sheet that you may use their email address to let them know about other Reiki events.

Operating a Reiki fundraiser will give you valuable experience and enhance your professional reputation. You will also have the satisfaction of helping a group you believe in at the same time you're helping those who receive your Reiki sessions. Once the event is over, you're likely to get people wanting to come to you for additional Reiki sessions. See The Saga of a Reiki Fundraiser on page 32 of the Spring 2007 issue of *Reiki News Magazine* for more information.

Holistic Fairs

Getting a booth at a holistic fair can be another effective way to promote your Reiki practice. Get several Reiki practitioners to help you. Take a Reiki table, a sign and plenty of business cards and flyers. Offer ten or fifteen- minute Reiki sessions for $10 and have three or more Reiki practitioners giving the sessions to each person. Create a sign-up sheet that includes the recipient's email address. It's possible to generate income at the same time you promote your Reiki business.

These are a few of the many ways you can promote your Reiki business. As you try these ideas, and especially if you follow the manifesting meditation practice in Part I of this series, you'll come up with additional ways that are just right for you. As you move forward and achieve your goal, you'll experience the miracle-working power of Reiki manifesting abundance in your life. Usui sensei said, "Reiki is the secret art of inviting happiness." Certainly you will experience a great happiness as you create a thriving Reiki practice. May you always be blessed by the radiant light of Reiki.

Creating a Reiki Class

Teaching Reiki classes can be very rewarding. Watching your students receive the ability to give Reiki for the first time can fill your heart with joy. Seeing their surprise and delight at the new energy they are experiencing, and then having them follow your guidance as they learn to give Reiki treatments to themselves and others is a meaningful experience. The advanced classes are even more fulfilling as your students will now have experience with Reiki and be excited about learning more or becoming Reiki Masters themselves. If you are a Reiki Master and have been hesitant to teach for whatever reason, I encourage you to move forward and plan to begin teaching; the rewards that come from teaching far outweigh the effort necessary to prepare or any concerns about the responsibilities that are required to do it well. Learning new skills and helping others are important parts of personal growth. By deciding to become a teaching Reiki Master and accepting this as an important part of your spiritual path, you will be propelled more quickly on your journey and experience greater fulfillment. Developing the skills necessary and working with your students will expand your comfort zone and enhance your self-worth. The appreciation and love you and your students develop for each other can affect you deeply and create memories that last a lifetime.

Outcomes

It's important to consider what can possibly take place in a Reiki class and in what way it can affect your students and yourself. A well organized and facilitated class, presented with love and compassion and balanced with the clear expression of factual information along with adequate demonstration and practice time can lift your students up to an entirely new level of awareness and self-esteem. If presented in this way, they will be motivated to use Reiki on themselves and others. Hopefully some will also consider eventually starting a Reiki practice of their own or becoming Reiki teachers so that the good you create in class will continue on as your students use Reiki to help and train others. With this in mind, a well-presented Reiki class can become a significant turning point in the lives of your students.

A student I will call Alice came to class because she was interested in learning about alternative healing, and a friend had mentioned Reiki to her. Having recently lost her job, Alice was collecting unemployment and had some free time. In class while practicing Gyoshi ho, she realized she was clairvoyant. This surprised her, as she had never thought of herself as psychic. After class she began giving free treatments to friends and found that many were enthusiastic about her Reiki. This inspired her to start a professional practice, and she eventually took the master training. The last I heard, she was teaching classes all over the Southwest. While Alice's story is exceptional, it is not unique. Reiki has changed the lives of many students.

Preparation

It is important that you have a well thought-out class outline and that you go over it and practice the meditations, demonstrations, discussions and exercises until you feel confident with them. Class outlines are on pp. 148.

It is even more important that you prepare your own energy. Being in a confident, optimistic, compassionate and supportive state of mind is necessary if one is to bring out the best in one's students. This most easily takes place when you are aligned with the Reiki consciousness. When in this state, the Reiki energy can surround you and move through you as you teach so that the thoughts and feelings you present become part of the flow of Reiki's expression.

This is a special kind of Reiki energy that is different than the energy that comes when we give Reiki sessions. I call this *teaching Reiki energy*, and it is an energy that works directly with the energy of the classroom and with each student, supplying each with what is needed to learn and to heal. Teaching Reiki energy can be cultivated by sending Reiki to the class starting weeks before it begins and saying prayers, asking that each student receives the healing in class that is exactly right for him or her and will learn what each needs to learn. Also as you pray, surrender the class to Reiki and ask that the only energies present in the class will be those decided on by God. Ask also that the attunements be very powerful and effective and that your talks and meditations will be guided by Reiki. Do this for each class you teach and over time, a much higher and more deeply healing energy will begin to be present in your Reiki classes.

When it comes to teach, it is important to turn the class over to the guidance of Reiki and allow Reiki to guide you and guide the energies of the class and how the class unfolds. When this happens, it will have a deeply meaningful effect that will touch the hearts of your students. By being aware of the unique needs of the class and by being open to Reiki's guidance, a class can take on a life of its own, often creating beneficial results that are wonderful and amazing.

Before you teach your first class as well as after you begin teaching, the responsibilities you will be required to take on will likely push on your unresolved issues and sometimes create uncomfortable feelings including worry, doubt, fear, tension or other similar feelings. Do not think this unusual. It is a natural part of doing anything new. This has happened to some extent to just about everyone who has taught Reiki. Be sure to take some time to meditate on your feelings and use your healing skills to treat them. Also, line up Reiki sessions with others. The opportunity to heal yourself more deeply is an important part of teaching Reiki. As you move forward with your plans and treat the issues that come up, things you were afraid to do will be transformed into enjoyable and satisfying activities.

Class Materials

A good class manual is a must. A well-organized class manual will not only make it easier for you to teach the class, but will also be appreciated by your students. It should contain a clear description of what Reiki is, how it works, what it can heal and how to use it. It should also contain diagrams or pictures of all the hand positions for treating self and others, and instructions on how to do the various techniques you will be teaching including how to give a complete treatment. You may want to include additional handouts of the Reiki symbols if it is a Reiki II class or higher, your lineage, and other material that you will be presenting. *Reiki, The Healing Touch* is a good manual to use for teaching Reiki I & II and of course you can use this manual for teaching the ART/Master class. You can purchase these manuals from our web store, www.reikiwebstore.com. If you buy five or more you'll get a 30% discount.

Creating Group Rapport

A Reiki class is actually a synergy of many things: the students, each of whom is unique, having differing backgrounds and reasons for attending, your own personality, training and experience, the Reiki energy itself and the way you allow it to present itself through you. Many things can take place, not all of which everyone will be conscious of, but with the right intention on your part and also by not getting in the way, a bonding and group rapport can develop that can be an important part of the learning and healing process.

It is important that the members of the class quickly develop a positive, connected feeling among themselves and with the teacher. When this happens, the students will feel safe. This will help them relax and be open and receptive to the new material and experiences they will be having. It will also help them open more fully to their own healing process. And it will also make your job as teacher easier. Rather than having to struggle to teach each person individually, based on his or her unique vibration, developing group rapport will allow you to work with the group as a whole. When group rapport has developed, understanding spreads through the class like a wave, and the students tend to reinforce and validate the learning process for each other.

Group rapport can develop by having the members of the class do things together. This is best done right at the beginning of class. To do this, you can have them do things like smudge each other, give each other short Reiki sessions, do grounding exercises with each other, do introductions while sitting in a circle, have them hug each other or conduct a meditation involving the flow of energy around the circle. (The Sufi greeting or any other type of group blessing is a nice way to create group rapport.) Use your imagination, and I'm sure you can think of other similar exercises to break the ice and get people connected with each other. Also remember that during the class, it will be the state of your consciousness that will have the most important effect on group rapport. Make sure you have an open, positive, uplifting regard toward your students and be looking for ways to support and validate them. An important goal is for your students to leave the class with a positive attitude toward each other, toward Reiki, and toward their ability to use it.

Western and Japanese Techniques

In a well thought out class, it is important that students understand the latest information about the history of Reiki and learn both Western and Japanese methods. The Western style introduced by Takata Sensei has value and focuses on the use of standard hand positions for each client. The original Japanese Reiki Techniques (JRTs) taught by Usui

142

Sensei make use of one's intuition and help the student create treatments that are specifically tailored to the individual needs of the client. The Western method is more left brained and based on following a set of rules or guidelines when giving sessions. The Japanese techniques are more right brained and help develop and use one's intuition. Both methods have value and when taught together, give the student a wide range of choices in the use of Reiki. The JRTs contain valuable techniques such as Gyoshi ho—a method of sending Reiki with the eyes, Koki ho—a method of sending Reiki with the breath, Kenyoku—a method for cleansing your energy field, and Byosen Scanning—a method for finding areas in the client that need Reiki. (A JRT training video and DVD is available, and many of these techniques are also described in *Reiki, The Healing Touch.*)

It is important to let the students know that Reiki cannot do harm and is actually quite flexible, and that there is no strict way that Reiki must be practiced. Encourage the students to trust in their own intuition and guidance when using Reiki and to discover those techniques they are most proficient with. By doing this, the students can develop a style based on their unique sensitivities and natural abilities. This is an important way for the students to advance as healers, which, in turn, will provide the greatest help to the client.

After Class Follow-up

Include enough practice time to give the students a feeling of confidence in the use of Reiki so that they will be inspired to use it on themselves and others after class. Continued practice is a must. To encourage this, have your students pick a Reiki buddy in class and have them agree to send distant Reiki to each other after class or to meet to exchange sessions with each other. You can also have each student commit to giving a certain number of treatments to family and friends. Organizing Reiki share nights are also important. At a share night, students can get together to share Reiki sessions with each other. This is a great service to your students, as some may not have anyone they can talk with about Reiki. The Reiki share group will be validating for them and will encourage them to continue using their Reiki abilities.

Conclusion

Creating a well organized and well taught Reiki class is a real service to individuals and to your community. It can also be a powerful part of your own spiritual path and contribute to your personal growth. As each of us accepts the challenges that are offered to us by our unique opportunities to serve others, our combined efforts are making a difference that will benefit ourselves as well as generations to come. May all you do be blessed by love.

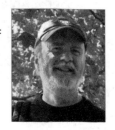

T HE ICRT REIKI MEMBERSHIP ASSOCIATION was created based on my twenty plus years of experience as a full time Reiki practitioner and teacher. Its purpose is to maintain a professional image for our members while at the same time preserving the spirit of Reiki and assisting members in creating a thriving Reiki practice. By becoming a member, you'll be associating with an organization that has the reputation of providing accurate, up-to-date information on the history, practice, and scientific study of Reiki. Our published, user-friendly membership list is an effective way to promote your sessions and classes. And our code of ethics and standards of practice allow those seeking a Reiki practitioner or teacher to know that choosing one of our members will result in a professional experience. An online database to keep track of your classes and students and class certificates that include both the name of your Reiki center (if you have one) and the membership association logo are available to Professional Members. We also have an amazing Reiki insurance policy available with a tremendous list of benefits and at a great price. To create community, we provide a social networking page for members to share experiences and ideas with each other and an online Reiki share group. It is my expectation that all our members will do well and to this end I'll be sharing my training and experience with you to ensure that every aspect of your Reiki practice is as professional and successful as possible.

Sincerely,

William Lee Rand

Membership is available to Reiki masters in the US or Canada.

Benefits of Joining the Reiki Membership Association

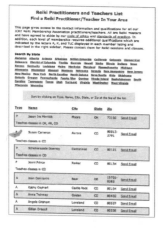

Advertise your Reiki practice

Being a member provides an effective way to promote your Reiki classes and sessions. One of the features of membership is a user-friendly searchable list of members that will allow those seeking Reiki sessions or classes to contact qualified Reiki practitioners and teachers. We promote this list on the reiki.org home page, which gets over 3000 visits a day, as well as in the *Reiki News Magazine*, our online newsletter, and other prominent places. This list is becoming the most popular list used by those seeking Reiki sessions or classes. Since launching the site in early January 2011, our Teacher/Practitioner page is already getting 400 visits a day by those looking for a Reiki practitioner or teacher. This service is included at no additional cost!

Keep Track of Your Classes and Students

A benefit for Professional Members is a secure online database that can be used to keep track of your classes and students. You'll be able to organize them by class, class type, last name, and zip code and also extract e-mail address lists. This service is included at no additional cost!

Print Student Certificates

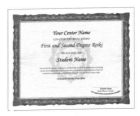

Another benefit for Professional Members is the ability to create Reiki class certificates online and download them to your printer. Certificates are printed instantly from our member web site and include your Reiki Center name (if you have one), the student's name, your name as the teacher, and will indicate your status as an ICRT Association Professional Member. A fee is charged for each certificate printed.

Membership Certificate

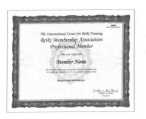

As soon as you join, you'll be provided with an ICRT Reiki Membership Association certificate that you'll be able to display on the wall of your Reiki room or show to prospective clients or students. This feature is included at no additional cost!

Social Network Group Page

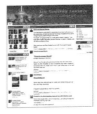

Members have exclusive access to our Group Page where you'll be able to post notices and share information with other members. This service is included at no additional cost!

Reiki Brochure

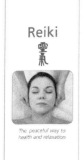

As a member you will be provided with a brochure to promote your Reiki business. This is a professionally produced brochure that clearly explains what Reiki is, how it works, what a session is like, and also provides scientific validation for its therapeutic value. The members' Reiki center (if you have one), your name, city, state, zip code, web site, e-mail address, and phone are automatically printed on the back by our computer program. This info can be edited by members to contain the information they want. They are downloadable from our web site so you can obtain them instantly and print them on their home printer. A version is also available for download that can be taken to a professional printer. The brochure is provided at no additional cost!

Reiki Insurance

A special Reiki insurance policy is available to our members. One policy covers Reiki and over 300 other modalities, including most forms of massage, bodywork, and energy therapy. It includes professional liability, general liability (slip and fall), classroom rental, lost or stolen equipment, product liability, and more! The policy follows you to wherever you practice or teach. Member price is only $149.00/yr.

Resources

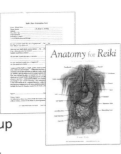

Our list of member resources includes: a Reiki exchange service that allows members to request distant Reiki for oneself, family, or friends; client documentation forms to help you keep track of your Reiki sessions; a full color "Anatomy for Reiki" chart; Reiki symbol handouts; and a list of articles to help you develop your Reiki practice, create a Reiki circle, learn how to work with animals, or provide Reiki for the terminally ill. We also include an article on how to get contact hours for CEUs set up for your students. In addition, you will be linked directly to our Reiki Research Center, which will keep you up-to-date on the latest scientific studies and provide valuable information and tools to help you get Reiki started in a medical setting. All of these resources are provided at no additional cost!

To learn more about our Reiki Membership Association and to join, please go to:

www.reikimembership.com

Values that Bring Success on All Levels

Reiki practitioners/teachers must allow themselves to conform to the nature of Reiki energy if they are to be perceived by others as authentic, and if they are to be truly successful. People cannot be easily fooled by surface spiritually now. They want the real teacher who comes from experience and is working on her or his own deep healing.

This is a continual process of working with all aspects of one's being that are out of step with Reiki, and allowing those aspects to heal. One must release all negative thoughts, feelings and energies as they arise, and allow the Reiki energy to replace them.

It is not wrong to have a negative thought or feeling, as we are all human. In fact, it is important for us to accept that we have faults and weaknesses. Only then can we release them into the Reiki Light to be healed.

The true nature of the Reiki energy is that it works in harmony with all people in a spirit of loving cooperation and free-flowing joy. True Reiki practitioners/teachers do not compete with others, but work in joyful cooperation. This means being happy about the success of others, even if we do not perceive ourselves as being successful.

In my experience, there have been two principles that have become the most important to me. They involve trust and humility and are as follows:

1. To trust completely in the God-Self or Higher-Power, as the only source of guidance and sustenance. Developed over time, with experience, this trust can become very effective. The God-Self knows everything about you and loves you completely. The God-Self is filled with complete wisdom and is all-powerful. You will never find a better source of help.

As your skill with Reiki grows, your personal power will grow as well. It is important that you never use your developing personal power to have power over others. If you are to be free and heal completely, it is important to use your increasing personal power to help others connect more strongly with the God-Self and to be free also. Do not compete with others, but become an increasing channel for the Divine Value the God-Self has to offer others through you. You have unique qualities and the Higher-Power has a special purpose for you that is different than anyone else. Focus only on allowing your Divine Purpose to shine forth and you will never have to worry about a lack of anything or about competition from others. In fact, after a while, you will realize that competition is only a figment of a negative imagination. It doesn't exist. Life is one flow of which we are all a part. Trust in the flow of life. Completely accept life. Allow life to flow through you to others. This is the way of Reiki. It will heal you in every way, bringing deeply felt happiness, peace and real freedom.

2. With humility, be willing to look at, feel, and release all impurity, negativity and darkness that is within you so that your true light will shine more brightly. Realize that your outer world is a reflection of your inner state. If there

146

are people or situations in your life that irritate you and that you don't like, then there will be a part inside of you of which you are mostly unaware that is also irritating and that you don't like. When you notice yourself having negative thoughts or feelings toward other people or situations, look inside yourself and be willing to accept that you attracted these people or situations into your life because they are similar to parts of yourself. Allow yourself to accept these parts of yourself. Ask to be shown the lesson they contain. Allow yourself to learn the lesson. Then forgive yourself and release the unbalanced part, the hurt part, into the Reiki Light. Let go of it and allow it to be healed. This is the mature way to deal with life's difficulties. As your inner self improves, so will your outer world. It takes courage and can also be painful, but as you do it, you will be building a foundation for success that can never be shaken. You will come to realize that all things in life have a place and are worthwhile and beneficial.

Class Outlines

The following class outlines are made available for your use. These are the class outlines used by the members of the Reiki Membership Association and by our Center Licensed Teachers. Feel free to teach exactly as outlined or to make changes to them. The outlines combine the Western style of Reiki with the Japanese style. The Reiki I & II outline is made to be used with the *Reiki, The Healing Touch* class manual, which includes instruction on how to do all the techniques in the outline including the Japanese Reiki Techniques (JRT). You may also want to get a copy of the Japanese Reiki Techniques Workshop DVD, which will instruct you on how to practice all the Japanese Reiki Techniques. The ART and Master outlines are to be used with this manual. These outlines are downloadable from our website.

Reiki I Training
Suggested class time: 9 a.m.–6 p.m.

1. Registration and sign in (required for CE providers).
2. Smudging (optional).
3. Introductions – name, work, family, metaphysical background, understanding of Reiki, why you want to learn Reiki, and something you like about yourself.
4. Opening meditation or prayer to join the group to the Higher Power and to each other.
5. Reiki Talk – what is Rei-ki? the different levels, how the attunement process works. How does Reiki work? (use information from the manual). What can it be used for? (Use examples and Reiki stories to explain these topics). History-Usui-Hayashi-Takata-22 masters, include info on the Gakkai and the discovery of the JRT techniques.
6. Lunch (one hour).
7. Return and regroup – circle shoulder massages and hugs.
8. Talk about attunement and how it works.
9. Explain Gassho meditation (page 54), and use this just before the attunement. Have students remain in Gassho during the attunement.
10. Reiki I attunement.
11. Have students write in their notebooks about attunement and meditation experiences—then share.
12. Break (10 minutes).
13. Practice Reiki (three or four to a group) – make sure all feel Reiki or that the client does. Share after.
14. Byosen Scanning (page 55) – pick a partner, scan, then switch. Explain Reiji-ho and that it is more advanced as one uses the intuition directly rather than the hand.
15. Explain and practice standard treatment, all hand positions (pick a partner and switch).
16. Explain and demo Kenyoku (page 59). Have students use it at end of treatment.
17. Explain *Hayashi Healing Guide* (page 63) and how to use it.
18. Explain client release forms and charging money or barter.

19. Break (10 to 15 minutes).

20. Explain self treatment – Byosen self scan (page 58) and practice self treatment hand positions.

21. *If students are continuing the next day: Reiki II Symbols – Show for memorization only, sacred, keep them secret, explain test. Distribute handout. (Use last 1/2 hour of class for this part.) If students are taking Reiki II, it's a good idea to give each a copy of the Reiki II symbols several weeks before the class so they have time to memorize them.

22. Closing meditation or prayer.

Reiki II Training
Suggested class time: 9 a.m.–6 p.m.

1. Sign in (required for CE providers) – Smudging (optional).

2. Opening meditation or prayer to join group to the Higher Power and to each other.

3. Sharing – meditation, effects from attunement, use of Reiki, questions or comments. Complete anything you did not have time for on Saturday (such as the self treatment).

4. Talk on Reiki II symbols – deeper, complete meaning, how to use them including the many ways to use Hon Sha Ze Sho Nen for distant and past/future healing.

5. Explain and demo Koki-ho (page 58). Explain and demo Jacki-Kiri joka-ho (page 60).

6. Lunch (one hour). Students can use some of their lunchtime to memorize the symbols.

7. Test on symbols – use form on page 157. If there are errors, gently point them out and ask student to correct them. Use hints if necessary or have the person use her notes. Coach so that everyone passes.

8. Circle massage and hugs.

9. Reiki II Attunement – include Gassho (page 54) at beginning.

10. Have students write attunement experiences in notebook – sharing.

11. Break (10 minutes).

12. Explain how to do complete treatment using all symbols.

13. Break up into groups of 3–4 to practice. Start with them doing straight Reiki without any symbols. Then have them add the Choku Rei and after five min. or so, share what this felt like. Do the same with the Sei heki so they get an experience of what the symbols do in class. Also, have them practice Koki-ho.

14. Practice Gyoshi-ho (page 60) – choose partners and switch. This can be done with the students sitting in two rows of chairs facing each other. Also explain that this can be done in regular treatment. (Note that this replaces Beaming.)

15. Enkaku chiryo (page 60) with group. Ask for requests from students. Write the names of those you are sending Reiki to on a piece of paper and place in the middle of the circle or use a photo of the person if it is available. Send to create harmony among all people on the planet, or perhaps a world situation. (World healing topics are located at www.reiki.org web site global healing network page.)

16. Have students pick a partner to exchange Reiki with during the week and send distant Reiki to.
17. Ending meditation and/or prayer.
18. Encourage students to participate in a Reiki support group.

Advanced Reiki Training Class (ART)
Suggested class time: 9 a.m.–6 p.m.

1. Registration and sign in
2. Smudging (optional).
3. Introductions – name, work, family, metaphysical background, understanding of Reiki, why you want to learn Reiki, and something you like about yourself.
4. Opening meditation or prayer to join the group to the Higher Power and each other.
5. Explain what the class will include, which parts are from Usui system and which parts are from the International Center for Reiki Training Research and Development.
6. Using crystals and stones with Reiki – how to use a single crystal to send Reiki continuously. Making a Reiki grid that will continue to send Reiki to yourself and others: used for distant healing, personal healing, goals and manifestation.
7. The Usui Dai Ko Myo – show it to students, explain usage, practice drawing it. Go over the meaning of the Japanese words and explain what it means to Reiki people.
8. Lunch (one hour). Use some of lunchtime to memorize symbol.
9. Test on symbol.
10. Explain how attunement works. That the attunement does not come from the teacher, but is channeled through the teacher in a similar way as the Reiki energy is channeled.
11. Advanced Reiki Attunement – explain and do Gassho (page 54) before and during attunement.
12. Moving Meditation.
13. If you have time, do "Meet Your Reiki Guides" meditation.
14. Write in notebook about attunement and meditation—then share.
15. Break (10 to 15 minutes).
16. Reiki Meditation – strengthens the mind and expands consciousness, helps discern the changes in the Reiki energy by invoking each symbol.
17. Reiki Aura Clearing (Psychic Surgery) – assists in removing negative psychic energy from yourself and others. Explain, demonstrate, and have students pick a partner and practice.

Use these steps if students are continuing the with the master training

20. Reiki Master Symbols – show for memorization only, sacred, keep them secret, explain test. Distribute handout. (Use last 1/2 hour of class for this part.)
21. Review Hui Yin exercise. Suggest that the students study and practice the Violet Breath exercise.
22. Closing meditation or prayer.

Reiki Master Class
Suggested class time: Two days from 9 a.m. – 6 p.m.

Day 1

1. Registration
2. Smudging (optional).
3. Introductions (for new people joining class only – name, work, family, metaphysical background, understanding of Reiki, why you want to learn Reiki, and something you like about yourself. Students who were in ART should tell new people their names and something about themselves.
4. Opening meditation or prayer to join the group to the Higher Power and each other.
5. Explain what the class will include for the two days, and which parts are from Usui system and which parts are from the Center for Reiki Training Research and Development.
6. Explain the Anthakarana. Suggest using it in class meditations and attunements by placing it under the chair or in front.
7. Review or explain the Hui Yin exercise if not covered in ART.
8. Microcosmic Orbit Meditation – explain and guide class (or use CD available from the Center), explaining the energy flow, and introducing the functioning and governing channel. This helps prepare the class for understanding the Violet Breath.
9. Optional – rather than do the Microcosmic Orbit Meditation, just explain how to do it. Then spend this time exchanging Reiki using the Usui Dai Ko Myo. Have 2–3 students give Reiki to one other. Sit in chairs or use Reiki tables. Take 5–10 minutes per person depending on the amount of time you have available.
10. Tibetan Symbols – show them to students, explain usage, practice drawing them.
11. Lunch (one hour). Use some of lunchtime to memorize symbols.
12. Test on symbol.
13. Explain how attunement works.
14. Reiki Master Attunement. Do Gassho (page 54) before and during attunement.
15. Write in notebook about attunement and meditation—then share.
16. Break (10 to 15 minutes).
17. Violet Breath – explain, demonstrate, have students practice.
18. Healing Attunement – explain, demonstrate and have students practice. One way to do this is for the teacher to demonstrate Part One. Then have the students break up into groups of three and have one sit in a chair and receive the Part One, have one do Part One and the other person can hold the manual and guide the one doing Part One. Then have each student rotate so each gets a change to practice, receive and guide. Do this with each part. Then have them practice all four parts at one time.
19. Have students do a complete Healing Attunement on each other with the purpose of healing an issue they have. Finish with Aura Clearing and Reiki if needed so that each receives a deep healing.
20. Questions and Answers.
21. Ask students to review the attunement for Reiki I and II as homework.

Day 2

1. Smudging (optional).
2. Opening meditation or prayer.
3. Discussion – the values and spiritual orientation of a true Reiki Master.
4. Practice Reiki I Attunement using same method as Healing Attunement – discuss, demonstrate, have students practice.
5. Lunch (one hour).
6. Questions and Answers.
7. Reiki II Attunement – discuss, demonstrate, have students practice.
8. Advanced Reiki Training Attunement – discuss, demonstrate, have students practice. (If students are feeling overwhelmed, demonstrate only.)
9. Reiki Master Attunement – discuss, demonstrate, have students practice.
10. Review differences in Usui attunement method – demonstrate Usui attunements. Have students practice the Usui attunements, but only if you have time and if the students have the energy to do so.
11. Explain self attunements and how to do the healing attunement at a distance. Explain that distant attunements are not as valuable as those done in person and only the healing attunement should be done at a distance.
12. Explain the need to practice and show how to practice on a teddy bear or pillow or on ones self by doing a self attunement.
13. Closing meditation and prayer and pass out class reviews.

Notes

Forms & Resources

Reiki Symbol Quiz

Teachers Name: _____ Class Date: _____

Class Location- City: _____ State: _____

What caused you to take this Reiki Class: (please circle all that apply)

reiki.org Internet site   Teachers personal internet site   Open House/Reiki Share

From a Friend   Reiki News   Other _____

Please Circle Class: Reiki II   ART   Master   Karuna I   Karuna II   Karuna Master

Student Name (please print) _____

Mailing Address: _____ City: _____

State: _____ Zip: _____ Country: _____

Phone number: _____ E-mail: _____

Please draw the symbols for this class level below and/or on the back without looking at your notes. Be sure to include the names of the symbols. The numbers and arrows are not necessary.

Anatomy *for* Reiki

ILLUSTRATIONS BY TOM BOWMAN

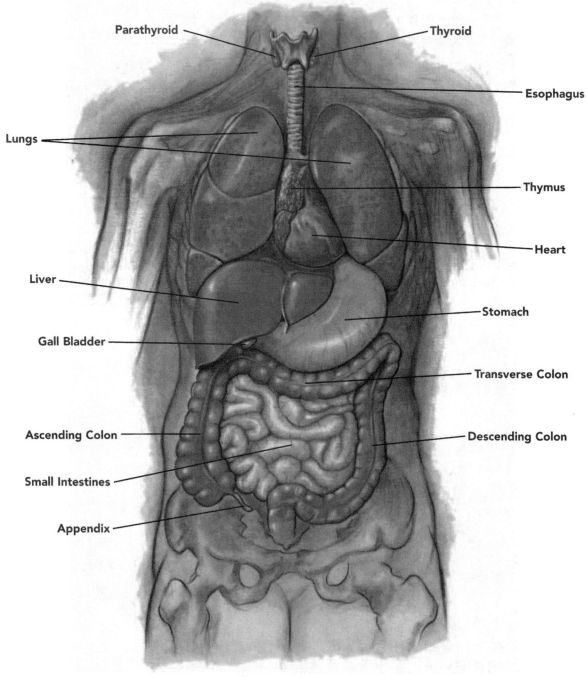

Parathyroid — Thyroid

Esophagus

Lungs

Thymus

Heart

Liver

Stomach

Gall Bladder

Transverse Colon

Ascending Colon

Descending Colon

Small Intestines

Appendix

Front View

While an extensive understanding of anatomy is not necessary for Reiki practitioners, there are times when a basic knowledge of the major organs of the body is helpful, and even necessary. These include when the client has a condition or illness involving a specific organ(s) that needs treatment or when working in a clinic or hospital where communication with medical personnel about a client's condition is necessary.

Adrenals: Part of the endocrine system, the adrenals secrete hormones that regulate various functions in the body, one of which is the flight or fight response.

Appendix: The appendix is located at the beginning of the colon on the lower right side of the abdominal cavity. It is medically said to have no function.

Colon: Consisting of the ascending, transverse, and descending sections, this tube-like organ is also called the large intestine and joins the small intestine on the lower right side of the abdominal cavity. The final processes of digestion take place in the colon with the absorption of water from fecal matter.

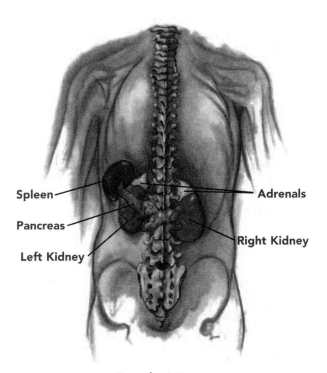

Spleen
Pancreas
Left Kidney
Adrenals
Right Kidney

Back View

Esophagus: The esophagus is the portion of the digestive tube that moves food from the mouth to the stomach.

Gallbladder: Connected to the liver, the gallbladder stores and secretes bile, which aids digestion of fats.

Heart: This is the muscular organ that pumps blood to all parts of the body. The rhythmic beating of the heart is a ceaseless activity, lasting from before birth to the end of life.

Kidneys: The purpose of the kidneys is to separate urea, mineral salts, toxins, and other waste products from the blood, and to conserve water, salts, and electrolytes.

Liver: The liver is the largest glandular organ of the body and has many functions including filtering debris and bacteria from the blood, converting excess carbohydrates and protein into fats, and producing blood-clotting factors and vitamins A, D, K, and B12. It also produces bile, which is used to prepare fats for digestion.

Lungs: The lungs are elastic organs used for breathing; they oxygenate the blood.

Pancreas: The pancreas is a glandular organ that secretes digestive enzymes and hormones. It also produces insulin, which lowers the blood-sugar level and increases the amount of glycogen (stored carbohydrate) in the liver.

Parathyroid: These four small glands are often embedded in the thyroid gland and govern calcium and phosphorus metabolism.

Small Intestine: Located between the stomach and colon, the small intestine digests and absorbs nutrients from food. This process is aided by secretions from the liver and pancreas.

Spleen: The spleen acts as a filter against foreign organisms that infect the bloodstream, and also filters out old red blood cells from the bloodstream and decomposes them.

Stomach: The stomach is the part of the digestive tract between the esophagus and the small intestine.

Thymus: The thymus gland helps in the development and functioning of the immune system.

Thyroid: Part of the endocrine system, the thyroid gland secretes hormones necessary for growth and metabolism.

Reiki Client Information Form

Name: (Please Print) _____

Phone (home): _____ Cell phone or evening: _____

Address: _____

City, State, Zip: _____

Email (optional): _____

Emergency Contact: _____

Current Medications and dosage: _____

_____

_____

Are you currently under the care of a physician? ___ Yes ___ No

If yes, physician's name: _____

How did you hear about us? _____

_____

Have you ever had a Reiki session before? ___Yes ___No

If yes, when was your last session? _____

Number of previous sessions _____

Do you have a particular area of concern? _____

_____

_____

Are you sensitive to perfumes or fragrances? _____

Are you sensitive to touch? _____

I understand that Reiki is a simple, gentle, hands-on energy technique that is used for stress reduction and relaxation. I understand that Reiki practitioners do not diagnose conditions nor do they prescribe or perform medical treatment, prescribe substances, nor interfere with the treatment of a licensed medical professional. I understand that Reiki does not take the place of medical care. It is recommended that I see a licensed physician or licensed health care professional for any physical or psychological aliment I may have. I understand that Reiki can complement any medical or psychological care I may be receiving. I also understand that the body has the ability to heal itself and to do so, complete relaxation is often beneficial. I acknowledge that long term imbalances in the body sometimes require multiple sessions in order to facilitate the level of relaxation needed by the body to heal itself.

Signed: _____ Date: _____

Privacy Notice:
No information about any client will be discussed or shared with any third party without written consent of the client or parent/guardian if the client is under 18.

Reiki Documentation Form

Client Name: _____ Date: _____

Reason for Session
___ Relaxation and Stress Reduction
___ Specific Issue:
     Physical_____
     _____

     Emotional _____
     _____

     Mental/Spiritual _____
     _____

Changes since last session: _____
_____
_____

Observation / Scan before Reiki Session:_____
_____
_____

Observation / Scan after Reiki Session: _____
_____
_____
_____

Post Session Notes: _____
_____
_____
_____
_____
_____
_____

Length / Type of Session:_____
Follow up Planned:_____
_____
_____

Practitioner Name: _____

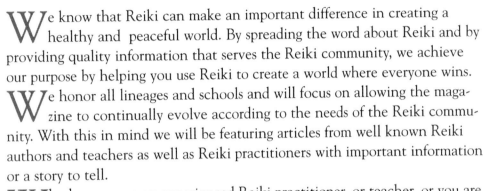

The Reiki Touch
A Tool Kit for Reiki Practitioners

The kit includes: DVD ~ Workbook ~ 2 CDs ~ Reiki Cards: $39.95

LAST YEAR THE PEOPLE AT SOUNDS TRUE contacted me about creating a Reiki multimedia instructional kit. I was very excited about the idea and in fact, I had already been thinking of doing something like this on my own. So we combined our resources and created a really wonderful package.

The audio was produced at their studio in Boulder, Colorado. The video portion was produced on a sound stage using a specially constructed set. A crew of ten was employed including a producer, director, and camera, sound and lighting people. Working with such a tightly focused group of professionals was a wonderful experience and I am very happy with the results.

This is my best work to date and includes ideas and techniques I've learned from others; developed on my own; and practiced and taught effectively over the course of 25 years. The basics of Reiki are clearly explained including the self-treatment, treating others, the symbols and sending Reiki at a distance. In addition, a number of the most advanced Reiki techniques have been included.

DVD

This one hour DVD includes the following:

TREATING OTHERS: Learn how to correctly give a complete treatment using all the standard hand positions. The glands, organs and chakras treated by each position are explained in detail.

SELF-TREATMENT: Follow along as I demonstrate the self-treatment — much like an exercise video. The glands, organs and chakras treated by each hand position are explained in detail and additional suggestions are included to increase the strength of your Reiki; help you relax more deeply; and improve the effectiveness of the treatment. This is an excellent way to learn the hand positions while at the same time giving yourself a treatment.

BYÓSEN SCANNING: A Japanese Reiki Technique, Byósen Scanning uses the sensitivity in your hands to discover where the client is most in need of Reiki. A demonstration and clear, straightforward instruction is included making it easy for anyone to learn this technique. An advanced method is also explained which combines Byósen Scanning with Gyóshi ho enabling the student to scan with the eyes.

GYOSHI HO: Another Japanese Reiki Technique, which involves sending Reiki with the eyes. This technique enables you to send Reiki to anyone you can see; such as a person on the other side of a room or outdoors and so forth. Gyoshi ho is an excellent technique for: treating children while they are playing, sending Reiki to various parts of your own body, or use it during a regular hands-on treatment to send additional Reiki where your hands are placed or to other areas.

SEEING AURAS AND PAST LIVES: This technique has been highly successful with over 95% of students getting results on the first try! Based upon Gyóshi ho, there are several reasons it works so well. First, because you are sending Reiki to the person's aura; Reiki strengthens their aura making it easier to see. Second, because you are sending Reiki with the eyes, the perceptive ability of the eyes merges with the higher dimensional nature of the Reiki energy thus raising the vibration of the eyes and making it possible to see the aura and past life imagery. The demonstration and clear instruction on this DVD make it easy to understand and get results. This technique can be used with a partner or with yourself while looking in a mirror.

ATTUNEMENT NECESSARY: The Reiki Touch kit is meant for those who have taken a Reiki class(s) and received an attunement, or who are planning to do so. The attunement is a necessary part of Reiki training and is best experienced in person from a qualified Reiki Teacher.

HEALING SESSION: At the end of the DVD, I beam Reiki directly to the viewer using my eyes and hands. By simply sitting in front of the screen you will receive a Reiki treatment.

REIKI CARDS

A set of 30 uniquely designed cards that demonstrate the Reiki hand positions, symbols (but not the glyphs), and proper Reiki techniques. Each card includes a detailed description. The cards can be used like flash cards to help you learn the various aspects of Reiki. They can also be used to do a Reiki card reading. By following the instructions, you will be able to use the cards along with the intuitive power of Reiki to guide you to the best hand position(s), symbol(s) or technique(s) to treat a specific issue – for yourself or others. So often when we are in need of healing, the stress of the situation inhibits our ability to call on the full range of healing tools and techniques we have available to us. The Reiki Cards allow you to call on higher wisdom to guide your use of Reiki. I have used my own home made version of these cards for years and it is uncanny how helpful and revealing they can be.

CD 1

This CD contains three Reiki meditations. As you listen to the meditations, you're asked to give yourself Reiki as you're guided into higher states of consciousness and offered new healing skills and energies. You will also be presented with the possibility of accepting an enlightened being as your personal guide. The first meditation increases the strength and effectiveness of your Reiki energy and deepens your healing process. The second creates a field of Reiki energy that surrounds you and protects you from all negative influence. The last meditation is for problem solving and creativity. The wonderfully soothing music of Nawang Khechog is played in the background of the meditations.

CD 2

This CD features background music to be played during Reiki treatments featuring the flute music of Nawang Khechog.

WORKBOOK

A 100-page workbook is included that contains detailed information on every aspect of Reiki from basic instruction to the most advanced techniques. Sample chapters include: What is Reiki?; How it Heals; History of Reiki; Symbols; Treating Self and Others; Research; Byósen Scanning; Gyóshi ho; Seeing Auras and Past Lives; Increasing the strength of your Reiki; Spiritual Protection; Reiki and Spirit Release; Creativity and Problem Solving; How to Receive Guidance from an enlightened being; Reiki and world peace, and more.

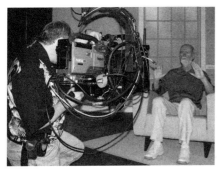
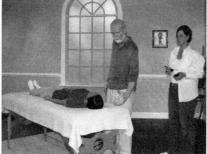
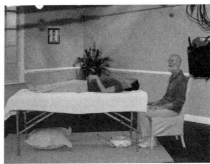

Reiki
The Healing Touch
First and Second Degree Manual

BY WILLIAM LEE RAND

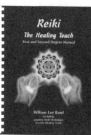

This book is a must for anyone wanting the latest information on Reiki. It includes discoveries about the roots of Reiki based on original documents and research in Japan. All the information in this manual has been researched and confirmed to be accurate! It also contains the most important of the Japanese Reiki Techniques taught by Dr. Usui and the Hayashi Healing Guide along with a method on how to combine them with the Western style of Mrs. Takata. Fully illustrated with more than 40 drawings and 18 photos

An excellent introduction to Reiki as well as a user-friendly manual for experienced practitioners.

- A clear explanation of Reiki
- How to use Reiki to heal yourself and others
- Includes all the hand positions
- Reiki symbols clearly explained
- Japanese Reiki Techniques
- Hayashi Healing Guide
- Becoming a Reiki Master
- Developing your Reiki practice
- Reiki in Hospitals
- Extensive footnotes and index

Used by over 4000 Reiki masters as their class manual.

Spiral bound so it lies flat
ISBN 1-886785031, 176 pages, 8-1/2" x 11"
Price: $19.95

Also available in perfect bound version
ISBN 1-886785058, 220 pages, 5-1/2" x 8-1/2"
Same information and price

Teacher Discount: Order 5 or more
of same book and get a 30% discount

Ask for these titles at your local bookstore, or order directly from: VISION PUBLICATIONS, Southfield, MI Toll Free 1-800-332-8112 or 1-248-948-8112 Order from our web site and get an additional 10% discount, www.reikiwebstore.com

Reiki In Hospitals PowerPoint Presentation

We've developed a Reiki in hospitals PowerPoint presentation to be shown to hospital administrators and staff that will help explain how a Reiki hospital program would work. It explains Reiki, includes Reiki research, explains the benefits of Reiki and the various types of Reiki programs hospitals are currently using, and also includes a list of prominent hospitals that have Reiki programs and so forth.

Table of Contents

Overview of Reiki
- What is Reiki? Fable vs Fact
- Reiki In Action

The Science of Reiki
- Brief overview of the Touchstone Project
- Major findings and conclusions

Overview of Reiki's Potential as an Offering in Hospitals and Clinics
- Hospitals that have started Reiki Programs
- Potential Benefits
- Examples of Outcomes
- Types of existing programs

Resources for building a hospital-based Reiki program
- Contact Information

$25.00

Download directly from our web site:
www.reikiwebstore.com

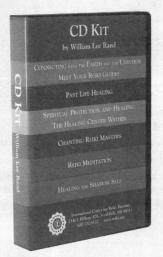
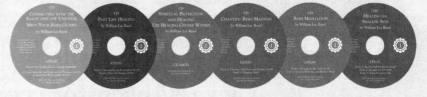
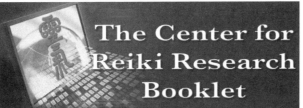
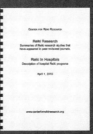
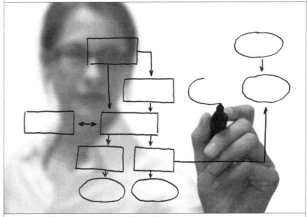
169

Developing Your Reiki Practice

An Anthology From *Reiki News Magazine*

This is an anthology of articles from the Reiki News written by people who have developed thriving Reiki practices. They explain what worked and what didn't work and what you need to do to make your Reiki business as successful as you'd like it to be.

Table of Contents

Create a Thriving Reiki Practice, Part I – Vision, Intention and Attitudes by William Lee Rand • **Create a Thriving Reiki Practice, Part II** by William Lee Rand • **Keys to a Successful Reiki Practice** by Particia Mahaffey • **Reiki Centers: How Seven Owners Achieved Success** by Patricia Mahaffey • **Starting a Reiki Practice: Business Basics** by Marianne Streich • **Creating a Reiki Circle for Your Community** by Elleen Dey, M.A. • **Creating A Successful Reiki Community "We" instead of "Me"** by Kimberly Fleisher, M.Ed • **Become an Approved Continuing Education Provider** by Dawn Fleming • **Secrets of a Traveling Reiki Master** by William Lee Rand

Phone: 1-800-332-8112 or 1-248-948-8112

Save 10% on most product orders completed on our website

www.reikiwebstore.com

An online digital version in color is also available for £8 (approx. $12.65).
Go to www.free.yudu.com, create your free account and search for reiki.

Notes